QUANTIFICATION OF CIRCULATING PROTEINS

Quantification of circulating proteins

Theory and applications based on analysis of plasma protein levels

by

WIM TH. HERMENS, GEORGE M. WILLEMS,
MARJA P. VISSER

Department of Biophysics, Biomedical Centre,
University of Limburg, Maastricht

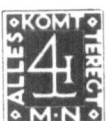

1982

MARTINUS NIJHOFF PUBLISHERS
THE HAGUE / BOSTON / LONDON

Distributors:

for the United States and Canada

Kluwer Boston, Inc.
190 Old Derby Street
Hingham, MA 02043
USA

for all other countries

Kluwer Academic Publishers Group
Distribution Center
P.O. Box 322
3300 AH Dordrecht
The Netherlands

Library of Congress Catalog Card Number: 82-19094

ISBN-13:978-94-009-7662-7   e-ISBN-13:978-94-009-7660-3
DOI: 10.1007/978-94-009-7660-3

PREFACE

Less than 50 years ago it was discovered that steady-state protein concentrations in plasma are the net result of continuous elimination and synthesis of protein molecules. The first quantitative studies on the turnover and distribution of plasma proteins were made around 1950, after the introduction of radiolabeled protein preparations.

Around 1970, another development in quantitative interpretation of circulating proteins was initiated in clinical enzymology. Estimation of cumulative release into plasma of cellular enzymes can be helpful in a variety of diseases to assess the extent of tissue damage and to evaluate therapy.

Enzymes can be considered as biological tracers, i.e. minute quantities of protein can be accurately determined by their specific catalytic activities. However, radioactive tracers permit direct estimates of turnover and distribution by measurement of excreted radioactivity, possibilities that are not available for enzymes. Consequently, only a few techniques used in tracer studies with radiolabeled proteins can be applied to circulating tissue enzymes and this may explain the lack of communication between the fields of plasma protein metabolism and quantitative clinical enzymology.

In the present study a summary is given of the basic methods used in both fields, with emphasis on the equivalence of various models and formalisms used by different authors. It is shown that major limitations in the study of circulating tissue enzymes can be overcome if two different, but simultaneously released, enzymes can be measured. The resulting method will also be applied to plasma protein metabolism.

Wim Th. Hermens, George M. Willems and Marja P. Visser

Maastricht, July 1982

CONTENTS

CHAPTER 1

INTRODUCTION

1.1 Quantitative description of circulating proteins

Circulating proteins as discussed in the present study gene-rally will be divided in circulating tissue proteins and plasma proteins. Circulating tissue proteins are present in plasma but have known biological functions outside the circulation. Examples of such proteins are intracellular contractile proteins like myosin or metabolic enzymes excreted into the gastrointestinal tract. The concentrations of these proteins in plasma are usually much lower than in tissues and their presence in plasma is con-sidered as the result of normal leakage of proteins from cells or as a sign of cell death. The large majority of circulating tissue proteins consists of enzymes that catalyse specific intracellular reactions. Therefore they may also be referred to as circulating tissue enzymes.

Proteins for which the presence in plasma is essential to their biological function are called plasma proteins. Classifi-cation is notoriously difficult because the biological function of many plasma proteins is not yet known [417,357]. Physico-che-mical characterization of these proteins is also hampered by the circumstance that some proteins are present in plasma in minute amounts and have only been discovered in relation to inherited protein deficiencies with well-defined clinical symptoms. Such accidental discoveries indicate the presence of many other un-known proteins.

Progress in the quantitative description of circulating tissue proteins and plasma proteins has been made along different lines and has provided answers to different questions.

Clinical enzymology originated with Wohlgemut, who developed a sensitive method for the determination of alpha-amylase in 1908 [535]. With this new assay he was able to demonstrate the presence of this tissue enzyme in serum and urine of patients with acute pancreatitis. Interest in this methodology was stimulated when, about 20 years later, the determination of alkaline phosphatase was introduced in the diagnosis of liver and bone disease [298,250]. The real break-through in this field came with the discovery in the fifties that acute myocardial infarction, as well as acute hepatitis, cause high plasma levels of aminotransferases ("transaminases") [269,536,133].

At that time the accuracy of enzyme determinations had sufficiently improved for a more quantitative approach. Several authors investigated the relation between plasma levels of cardiac enzymes and morphologically assessed infarct size after experimental myocardial infarction in dogs. Cumulative tissue damage can be accurately estimated in the heart because there is no regeneration of irreversibly damaged cardiac muscle cells. Also, the exact moment of onset of necrosis can usually be estimated in the clinical situation. For the liver, which is the most intensely studied organ in clinical enzymology, both these conditions are not fulfilled and attempts at quantitative interpretation of hepatic enzyme release have generally been inconclusive [411]. In the dog, a correlation between maximal plasma levels of cardiac enzymes and myocardial tissue injury was indeed found but this correlation was too low to allow accurate estimation of tissue damage from maximal plasma levels of aspartate aminotransferase and lactate dehydrogenase [5,334]. Still, a quantitative relation between enzyme release and tissue damage was again suggested when, a few years later, a highly significant relation was demonstrated between maximal levels of cardiac enzymes in plasma of patients with acute myocardial infarction and mortality as well as the incidence of cardiac failure [390,434,255].

In the mean time, quantitative methods for the study of circulating proteins were rapidly advancing in a field which has traditionally few links with clinical enzymology, i.e. the study of turnover and distribution of plasma proteins. The introduction of techniques for the labeling of proteins with radioactive isotopes in the fourties and fifties had triggered the study of in vivo elimination of injected protein preparations. Although

the initial results obtained from such experiments were contradictory due to a number of artefacts, such as re-utilization of
label or self-irradiation damage of proteins, these complications
were soon recognized and experimental procedures were corrected
accordingly. This resulted in a multitude of methods and models .
Some of these were based upon exponential analysis of disappearance curves from plasma after intravenous injection of labeled
protein preparations. Others made use of the possibility of
directly estimating catabolic rate constants by measuring the
rate of excretion of radioactivity in urine and faeces. Another
specific advantage of radiolabels is the possibility of direct
determination of the extravascular protein pool. To this end the
plasma pool, obtained from the plasma concentration of radioactivity and plasma volume, is subtracted from the total body pool
of protein as estimated by whole-body counting techniques or by
measuring cumulative excretion of radioactivity. Much information
was also obtained from observation of the behaviour of injected
synthetic macromolecules and the protein content of interstitial
fluid and lymph. In the sixties consistent data had been obtained
on the magnitude of intra- and extravascular protein pools,
mechanisms of transcapillary protein escape and pathways of
extravascular protein transport [417].

Partly as a result of this work on plasma proteins it was
realized that maximal levels of tissue enzymes in plasma do not
allow an accurate estimate of the quantity of enzyme released
into plasma under pathological conditions. Such maximal levels
are dependent on (biological variation in) the rate of catabolic
removal of enzyme from the plasma and on the rates of extravasation and extravascular return of protein. Due to these factors,
maximal levels of tissue enzymes in plasma are strongly influenced by the time-course of enzyme release. Release of short
duration causes higher maximal levels than release of the same
quantity of enzyme in a longer period of time. About 1970 the
quantitative relation between myocardial enzyme release and
cardiac damage was again investigated, and allowance was made for
elimination of enzyme from plasma and for specific features of
the circulatory model [530,424]. Subsequently, quantitative

interpretation of tissue enzyme levels in plasma has been applied in widely different fields such as evaluation of therapeutic interventions after acute myocardial infarction [299], comparison of techniques for protection of myocardium during cardiac surgery [116], prediction of rejection crises after organ transplantation [326,17], determination of platelet survival times [448], estimation of adaptation of athletes to prolonged excercise [45], determination of intralobular localization of liver damage [180] etc.

These examples illustrate the practical importance of accurate quantification of circulating tissue enzymes. However,many of the values of catabolic rate constants and rate constants for the transfer between plasma and interstitium of circulating tissue enzymes are known only approximately and less exact than similar values for plasma proteins. This is not caused anymore by a poor accuracy of enzyme determinations compared to the high accuracy of detection methods for radiolabeled proteins. Experimental scatter in enzyme determinations has been considerably reduced in the last decade, as shown by the successful competition between immuno-enzymatic assays and traditional radio-immuno assays. However, the analysis of circulating tissue enzymes is subject to other limitations. Many authors consider tissue enzymes as foreign elements in plasma and hesitate to inject such enzymes in patients because of the immunological risks. This eliminates the possibility of studying the effects of intravenous injection of enzymes in patients. Moreover, there are no direct methods for estimation of extravascular enzyme pools or excretion of enzyme degradation products as described for radiolabeled plasma proteins. Some authors have attempted to use transient release of tissue enzymes into plasma, e.g. during acute hepatitis, as a substitute for intravenous injection. Catabolic rates were estimated from the disappearance of enzymes from plasma during recovery. Such attempts resulted, however, in underestimates of the catabolic rates, because the duration of enzyme release was generally underestimated. This problem cannot be solved simply by taking a safety time-margin because most enzymes are rapidly eliminated from plasma and the rate of disappearance can only be determined during a short time interval.

A recently introduced method is based on the release of two different tissue enzymes, also in patients with acute tissue damage [527,528]. If both enzymes are released simultaneously, the catabolic rate constants can be determined even during continuous release. This method can also be applied to parallel changes in the rate of synthesis of two different plasma proteins. Circulatory parameters can thus be determined by the use of natural changes in plasma protein levels, instead of by injecting radiolabeled protein preparations. Applications of this method, both to circulating tissue enzymes and plasma proteins, will be presented.

1.2 Presentation of theory and applications

Quantification of circulating proteins is not always dependent on detailed knowledge of the circulatory model. If the rates of protein elimination and protein transfer are proportional to the quantities of protein, i.e. a so-called linear circulatory system, all information required for quantification of protein release in plasma can often be obtained from the plasma disappearance curve after an intravenous bolus injection of protein. This fact will be further illustrated in Chapter 4. However, quantitative studies on circulating proteins have always been closely connected to the specific physiological properties of the circulatory system. To determine such properties has been the primary purpose rather than to estimate the circulating quantities of protein. The use of specific physiological models has the advantage that previously obtained knowledge can be incorporated. For example, the magnitude of an extravascular protein pool can be estimated from the independent measurements of interstitial fluid volume and protein concentration in lymph. Interpretation of changes in plasma protein levels may be dependent on specific physiological information, e.g. the rate of protein synthesis can be measured in vivo from incorporation of radiolabeled amino-acids. The usual interpretation of such experiments, however, is dependent on the assumption that protein molecules enter the plasma directly after synthesis, and not after previous mixing with extravascular protein pools.

In view of this relation between physiological data and interpretation of plasma protein levels, Chapters 2 and 3 are devoted to physiological data relevant to the quantitative description of respectively circulating tissue enzymes and plasma proteins. Particular attention will be paid to the pathways of protein entrance, the distribution of proteins between intra- and extravascular protein pools and the mechanisms of protein elimination from the circulation. The biological variation in tissue enzyme content and the physiological significance of cellular leakage of proteins will be discussed in Chapter 2. Chapter 3 further contains a survey of the biological variations in the circulatory parameter values in man.

Chapter 4 contains a review of the methods applied for quantitative analysis of plasma protein levels. Although the equivalence of various methods is stressed, a variety of models and formalisms is discussed and this chapter may seem confusing. In that case it is advised to omit this chapter at first reading and to consider it as reference material. Mathematical expressions as used in Chapter 4 are carefully explained and it is expected that the average reader interested in medicine and physiology will be able to follow the discussion. For practical use of this chapter an appendix has been added containing some essential derivations of mathematical expressions, mostly by applying Laplace-transformations.

Artefacts which may occur in quantitative studies of circulating proteins are considered in Chapter 5. As an aid for the detection of such errors, a table is presented that contains the range of biphasic disappearance curves compatible with physiological data. This chapter also contains a section on errors in the calculated cumulative release of proteins in plasma. It is shown that such errors may be dominated by uncertainties in the value of a single parameter, e.g. biological variation in the fractional catabolic rate constant.

Chapters 6, 7 and 8 contain applications of various methods, both to estimation of enzyme release after tissue damage and to calculation of circulating mass of plasma proteins.

In Chapter 6 the problem is discussed of assessment of myocardial damage from plasma levels of cardiac enzymes. Catabolic rate constants of several enzymes can be obtained from analysis of time-activity curves in plasma of simultaneously released enzymes in patients with acute myocardial infarction. On the basis of this information it can be determined for which enzymes an accurate calculation can be made of the cumulative release. After cardiac surgery, the situation is complicated by enzyme release due to skeletal muscle damage and due to hemolysis. It is shown that these different forms of tissue damage may be separately estimated by use of appropriate combinations of enzymes.

Chapter 7 is devoted to the acute phase response, i.e. the general response to trauma with significant changes in the circulating mass of a number of plasma proteins like haptoglobin and C-reactive protein. The catabolic rate constants of these so-called acute phase reactants can be obtained from simultaneous measurement of fibrinogen levels. It is shown that changes in the rate of synthesis of different acute phase reactants are parallel.

Quantitative description of plasma levels of blood coagulation factors is discussed in Chapter 8. These proteins are infused in patients with inherited protein deficiencies and this has produced much information on plasma disappearance curves of coagulation factors. A practical problem in the treatment of such patients is to determine the required doses of protein needed for infusion in different situations, e.g. a single dose needed in acute events, maintaining of a high plasma level of coagulation factor by continuous or repeated infusion during therapeutic interventions such as surgery, or a relatively low but steady plasma level in prophylaxis. Some tables are presented, which can be used for dose-calculation in these clinical situations.

Chapter 9 contains a compilation of circulatory parameters as reported in literature for circulating tissue enzymes as well as for plasma proteins. This compilation actually is a critical review; many results presented in the literature have been omitted on account of possible errors as discussed in Chapter 5, or because the applied circulatory models proved to be unsuitable. However, excellent studies may have been missed because the literature in the fields of clinical enzymology and plasma protein metabolism is so comprehensive that completeness can hardly be attained. Moreover, new results are regularly published, e.g. for plasma lipoproteins and for the elimination mechanisms of glycoproteins.

Acknowledgements

The present study received its first impulse in 1969 in the department of Cardiology, University of Leiden, when Dr H.C. Hemker initiated a quantitative study of plasma enzyme levels in patients with acute myocardial infarction. The results were published as a Ph.D. thesis by Dr S.A.G.J. Witteveen [531]. In the following years a succesful cooperation came about between the departments of Biophysics and Biochemistry of the Medical Faculty at Maastricht and the department of Cardiology at Leiden. We are greatly indebted to Dr A. van der Laarse and Mrs L. Hollaar of the department of Cardiobiochemistry, Academic Hospital, Leiden for many years of stimulating collaboration. Data from patients as presented in Chapter 6 were obtained in this period. Changes in plasma levels of acute phase reactants, as presented in Chapter 7, were kindly provided by Dr S.J. Smith formerly at the department of Internal Medicine of the Medical Faculty at Rotterdam. The excellent medical records of Professor E.A. Loeliger at the department of Hematology, Academic Hospital, Leiden, proved to be indispensable in the search for plasma disappearance curves of blood coagulation factors as discussed in Chapter 8. Mrs F. Lakmaker, who spent much effort in screening the literature, has also produced the figures. Mrs R. Borgman-Hanssen never tired of retyping the manuscript and skilfully completed the final version.

PART A

Physiological basis, choice of models

and quantitative methods.

CHAPTER 2

TURNOVER AND DISTRIBUTION OF CIRCULATING TISSUE ENZYMES.

2.1 Introduction

Quantification of circulating proteins invariably concerns estimating quantities of protein entering and leaving the circulation in a certain period of time. In order to obtain such estimates, some properties of the circulatory system and of the specific protein have to be known. In some cases the information needed may be limited. For example, information on the fractional catabolic rate constant (FCR) and the plasma concentration of protein would be sufficient for calculating the amount of protein entering the bloodstream per litre of plasma per hour. However, often more information is needed. To estimate the amount of an enzyme leaking during necrosis from a damaged organ, a number of points have to be considered. First, the route of entrance into the circulation must be determined, and also possible inactivation of enzyme during transport from organ to plasma; further, the number of compartments in which the enzyme is distributed and the rates of exchange of enzyme between these compartments. Last but not least, for each of these compartments it must be ascertained whether enzyme inactivation takes place and at which rate. As there are obviously many compartments, these points require a great deal of information. It will be clear that quantitative estimates of circulating enzymes can only be made if part of this information can be discarded as irrelevant. Such a reduction of required information occurs for instance if the enzyme is known to be inactivated only intravascularly.

In Chapter 4 it will be discussed which information remains essential for computing circulating quantities of protein. In the present chapter and Chapter 3, the available information will be considered, i.e. a summary will be made of the main facts and hypotheses about entrance, distribution and elimination of pro-

teins in the circulation. In addition the question will be raised
whether release of tissue enzymes into the plasma can be quantitatively related to tissue injury. Attempts to answer this question have provided a large part of the data to be discussed. Some
authors have also studied the relation between tissue damage and
leakage of non-enzymatic cellular proteins such as myosin [481]
and myoglobin [509,454]. The present chapter will however mainly
be focussed on cellular enzymes.

2.2 Variability of tissue enzyme content.

A first question in the quantitative interpretation of release
of tissue enzymes in various diseases is whether plasma levels
measured in different patients can be compared. As it is practi-
cally impossible in most clinical cases to obtain individual
estimates of tissue enzyme content, comparison between individuals is possible only if we can use a fixed mean value for this
quantity, i.e. if variation between individuals in tissue enzyme
content is small. Moreover, it must be assumed that variation of
enzyme content between different sites of the damaged organ is
small also, unless the exact location of the injury within the
organ is known. The validity of both conditions will be investigated in the present section by considering data from the literature on inter- and intra-individual variation of tissue enzyme
content.

Absolute values of tissue enzyme content as mentioned by
various authors can hardly be compared. Activities are often
related to wet weight of tissue or to tissue protein content, dry
weight, total DNA or nitrogen content. Next to these different
ways of expressing the enzyme content of tissues, large differences in measured enzyme activities are introduced by variable
assay conditions such as temperature, pH, kind of substrate,
substrate concentrations, period of incubation or presence of
various "activators". Some of these differences are shown in
Table 2.1. They are cumbersome but do not present a serious
problem as long as each author mentions some standard reference
value, e.g. the activity determined in pooled normal plasma.

More important than differences in absolute (mean) values of tissue enzyme content are differences in reported variability. Earlier studies mentioned coefficients of variation (CV), i.e. standard deviations expressed as a percentage of the mean, as large as 31% and 27% respectively for the LDH* and AST* content of dog heart [179], 23% again for the LDH content of dog heart [286] or 36% and 48% for the LDH content of rat and mouse heart [148]. As mentioned in one of these previous studies [148], the apparent biological scatter in tissue enzyme content was of the same order of magnitude as the scatter inherent in the assay procedures available at that time. Considering the multitude of factors affecting enzyme determinations it is not surprising that gradual improvement and standardization of assay conditions led to steadily decreasing variability in the last 10-20 years. Use of commercially available "optimised" test kits has greatly contributed to this development. For this reason, Table 2.1 contains recently obtained results. As a number of additional errors is involved in isoenzyme separation, only values for total enzyme content are given.

A factor leading also to erroneously high variability of tissue enzyme content is the intracellular compartmentalization of enzymes. For instance for AST a large part of enzyme activity in heart and liver is located in the mitochondria (mAST). If cellular compartments are not properly disrupted, e.g. by sonification or use of detergents, variable fractions of mAST will not be liberated. For CK this phenomenon has caused errors in the quantity of heart-specific isoenzyme CK(MB) as determined with immunological assays. Varying quantities of mitochondrial CK were falsely considered as CK(MB) [525].

Another factor of importance in the determination of tissue enzyme content is sample size. The lower limit for detection of tissue damage from elevation of plasma enzyme levels is approximately 0.1-1 gram wet weight of tissue. Human tissue samples used

---

* cf. enzyme abbreviations in Table 9.6

for determination of tissue enzyme content are however usually biopts of 10-50 mg. Apart from increasing experimental error due to manipulation of samples, the use of small samples will tend to increase observed variability due to structural inhomogeneities such as vessel walls or connective tissue and due to the existence of mixed cell populations such as hepatocytes and Kupffer cells in the liver. For instance, a considerable inhomogeneity was found for the GLDH content of human liver using a microdissection technique and samples of 20-40 ng of dry weight [180].

The existence of mixed cell populations is also relevant to the relation between released quantities of tissue enzymes and loss of tissue mass. It has been demonstrated that shifts in myocardial enzyme content, traditionally interpreted as shifts in enzyme content of myocytes due to ageing or to increased energy demand, are caused by proliferation of fibroblasts [489,377]. In hypertrophic hearts, for instance, this finding would imply that loss of myocardial mass is underestimated if tissue damage is determined from plasma levels of enzymes which are virtually absent in fibroblasts such as CK. In cases of congestive liver damage, cell death occurs preferentially in the central zone of the liver lobules which are relatively rich in GLDH [180]. So loss of liver mass would be overestimated if it is determined from plasma levels of GLDH and an overall mean value of liver GLDH content.

These examples demonstrate the inherent difficulties in relating enzyme release from a damaged organ to histologically assessed tissue injury. Staining techniques, such as the well known method based on nitro blue tetrazolium (NBT), are unable to detect a small percentage of viable cells in a necrotic zone or a small fraction of dead cells in an otherwise undamaged area. Moreover, quantitative histologic methods have a considerable experimental error which may also cause poor correlation with enzymatic estimates of injury. The same is true for determination of tissue damage from ultrastructural changes as determined by electron microscopy. Features of increasing tissue injury such as disappearance of glycogen granules, mitochondrial swelling and disarray of mitochondrial cristae and myofibrils, are generally correlated to other measures of tissue damage [128,315]. However, no sharp "point of no return" can be determined and striking discrepancies between functional, ultrastructural and metabolic state have been observed [406]. To circumvent such problems, tissue damage has been simply defined by the loss of enzymes from the damaged organ in a number of studies [381,206,83].

Data on enzyme content of tissues obtained at autopsies should be considered critically because varying degrees of autolysis may result in overestimating variability. In 14 human myocardial autopsies CV of 17%, 16% and 8.6% were found for CK, AST and HBDH [492]. The remarkable stability of HBDH has been confirmed in a study demonstrating a CV of 7.3% for HBDH content of myocardium obtained from patients up to 36 hours after death, compared to CV of 21% for AST and 31% for CK [203]. In this respect the iso-enzymes LDH_1 and LDH_2 in heart tissue, which are measured in the HBDH assay, behave strikingly different from the isoenzymes LDH_5 and LDH_4 in skeletal muscle which are rapidly inactivated after death [408]. Even data obtained from human biopsies should be considered carefully because such data are usually obtained from patients and variability can be overestimated as the result of degenerative changes in tissue enzyme content.

Table 2.1 shows that significant regional differences in enzyme content exist in some tissues. Such variations are to be expected if functional differences exist between different re-gions in the organ such as found between kidney cortex and me-dulla or between different parts of the intestinal tract [413]. For skeletal muscle also significant differences in enzyme con-tent of fast-twitch (type I) and slow-twitch (type II) muscle fibres have been demonstrated [172,478]. The existence of trans-mural gradients of enzyme activity in the heart is also subject of controversies between earlier and recent work. A report on higher epicardial oxygen tension and blood flow [256] was supple-mented with the finding of higher glycogen levels at the endocar-dium of several species [232]. Subsequently it was reported that 5 out of 8 glycolytic enzymes, including LDH, showed elevated endocardial levels in dog heart [286], while indicators of oxida-tive metabolism such as the succinate-cytochrome C reductase

Table 2.1. Variability of tissue enzyme content

Species	Tissue	Enzyme	Expression of activity in U per gram of	Mean value (U)*	Temp. (°C)	Coefficient of variation between sites	Coefficient of variation between individuals (number of individuals)	Ref.
man	heart (left ventricle)	LDH	protein	1138	25		9.4 (8)	[492]
		LDH	wet weight	128	25		12 (15)	[532]
		HBDH	protein	903	25		11 (8)	[492]
		HBDH	wet weight	118	25		7.3 (12)	[203]
		CK	protein	6357	30		14	[492]
		CK	wet weight	370	25		10 (8)	[532]
		AST	protein	1067	25		11 (8)	[492]
		GPI	wet weight	143	25		10 (15)	[532]
	liver (different lobes)	LDH	protein	1453	25		12 (16)	[412]
		AST	wet weight	83	25	5.8	10 (15)	[412]
		AST	wet weight	83	25	3.1	18 (15)	[412]
	skeletal muscle different muscles	LDH	wet weight	377	25		11 (9)	[538]
		CK	wet weight	2071	30		31 (9)	[538]
	quadriceps	CK	wet weight	5250	37	4.3	15 (8)	[188]
	quadriceps	GPI	wet weight	380	37		21 (8)	[188]
	diafragm	CK	wet weight	3612	37	3.8	26 (9)	[40]
	rectus abdominus	CK	wet weight	4812	37		18 (10)	[40]
	kidney glomeruli	LDH	dry weight	635	37		34 (9)	[141]
	glomeruli	AST	dry weight	104	37		28 (4)	[141]
	glomeruli	AP	dry weight	9.3	37		13 (6)	[141]
	medulla	LDH	dry weight	1406	37		32 (6)	[141]
	medulla	AST	dry weight	335	37		18 (4)	[141]
	medulla	AP	dry weight	47.3	37		10 (6)	[141]

Table 2.1 (continued)

blood-cells									
erythro-cytes	LDH	hemoglobin	200	37		13	(10)	[54]
	LDH	U/10^{11} cells	329	25		7.6	(7)	[213]
	MK	hemoglobin	258	37		11	(10)	[54]
thrombo-cytes	LDH	U/10^{11} cells	150	25		27	(7)	[213]
granulo-cytes	LDH	U/10^{11} cells	10029	25		17	(7)	[213]
dog heart (diffe-rent ven-tricles)	CK	wet weight	3583	37	2.5	6.9	(10)	[505]
	LDH	wet weight	313	25	2.6	7.5	(10)	[505]
	AST	wet weight	181	25	3.0	12	(10)	[505]
	GPI	wet weight	165	25	2.5	5.6	(10)	[505]
liver (different lobes)	ALT	wet weight	88	25	1.8	11	(10)	[505]
	AST	wet weight	111	25	1.7	12	(10)	[505]
	GPI	wet weight	113	25	1.0	17	(10)	[505]
rat heart apex	LDH	wet weight	429	25		13	(15)	[531]
apex	CK	wet weight	414	25		14	(15)	[531]
apex	GPI	wet weight	98	25		6	(15)	[531]
pig heart left-ventricle	HBDH	wet weight	179	25	7.8	10	(11)	[203]
	CK	wet weight	982	30	5.8	13	(11)	[203]
	AST	wet weight	120	25	4.6	7.4	(11)	[203]
cow heart left-ventricle	LDH	protein	5747	25		8.5	(8)	[205]
	CK	protein	2442	25		18	(8)	[205]
	AST	protein	1235	25		14	(8)	[205]

*Enzyme activity is expressed in international units (U). One U of activity catalyses the conversion of 1 micromole of substrate per minute at indicated temperature and assay conditions.

system were found to be elevated in the subepicardium of bovine hearts [480]. From these data a picture emerged of a relatively hypoxic endocardium with a high work load and a high capacity for anaerobic glycolysis. This picture is not confirmed, however, by a number of recent studies. In hypertrophied and normal rat left ventricle no significant difference between endo- and epicardial LDH content was found [140], which was confirmed for dog heart [505]. Measurement of the deformation of canine myocardium during the cardiac cycle revealed a torsion of the left ventricle which minimizes the differences between endo- and epicardial work load [21,22]. It was also reported recently that in the normal working dog heart no transmural gradients in oxygen tension exist [487].

The figures presented in Table 2.1 also reflect variability due to experimental scatter in enzyme determinations and due to sample handling. Even in the simple case of enzyme activity expressed per gram wet weight of tissue, experimental error is at least 5%. After subtracting this error from the figures, it may be concluded that true variation between individuals for heart and liver enzyme content cannot be more than 5-10%. Thus, the use of fixed mean values for the tissue content of some diagnostically important enzymes will not introduce errors exceeding 5-10% in estimates of loss of tissue mass.

A significant fraction of the enzymes in healthy tissue is not released after injury. It was demonstrated that 48 hours after experimental myocardial infarction in dogs, tissue activity of the cytoplasmic enzymes ALD, GAPDH, LDH and GPDH in the central infarcted area was 19-25% of normal, whereas the enzymes MDH and AST, with large mitochondrial isoenzyme fractions, had decreased to respectively 35% and 47% of normal values [179]. The latter percentage confirms earlier figures on AST depletion of myocardium after infarction [334,325]. In contrast to MDH and AST, the mitochondrial enzymes ICDH(NAD) and succinate dehydrogenase do not show inhibited release after tissue injury. Rapid depletion and early release into plasma have been demonstrated for both enzymes after experimental myocardial infarction [179,455,233]. The best-documented enzyme in this respect is CK. Data on dog [206,424,381], man [61] and rabbit [257] show that within 24-48 hours after occlusion the CK-content of infarcted left ventricular tissue has decreased to 15-30% of normal values. More rapid washout of LDH, AST and succinate dehydrogenase to about 30% of initial values in 5-10 hours has been reported for the posterior papillary muscle in infarcted dog hearts [233].

The simplest explanation for the remaining enzyme activity in infarcted heart muscle would be the survival of 20-30% of myocytes in the necrotic zone. Indeed it has been shown by a variety of techniques that there is some remaining blood supply even in the central infarcted area. In one of these studies, however, it was shown that correction for "normally perfused" myocardium still leaves a figure of 20-30% of normal values for the CK content of the remaining necrotic tissue [206]. Apart from survival of myocytes, other factors such as retention of mitochondrial isoenzyme fractions, recruitment of blood cells, and proliferation of fibroblasts, must play a role. The importance of the latter factors is also suggested by the finding of a large increase of G6PDH and GPDH activity and changes in isoenzyme patterns during tissue repair [179,377]. Again one is confronted with difficulties in relating enzyme depletion to histological measures of tissue injury.

2.3 Relation between leakage of cellular enzymes and cell death.

Release of cellular protein is obviously a normal physiological function for cells producing export proteins. However, the diagnostic use of elevated plasma levels of tissue enzymes as a sign of tissue damage, initiated a discussion about the physiological significance of cellular leakage of enzymes which only have intracellular functions. The usual textbook on clinical enzymology states that depletion of cellular energy stores results into leakage of intracellular enzymes. Although this is certainly correct, the question whether cells could loose enzymes in normal physiological conditions remains unanswered. In fact this question has been debated during more than 50 years now, but no generally accepted answers have been given.

A number of studies deal with the relation between high energy

phosphates and irreversible cell injury in the ischemic or hypoxic heart. In a review [234] it is concluded that necrosis starts
when ATP levels have fallen to about 20% of the normal levels.
Roughly a similar relation is found between ATP-depletion and
onset of enzyme leakage from cultured beating fetal mouse and
chicken heart cells after inducing hypoxia [130]. It should be
noted, however, that ATP levels on itself need not give a correct
impression of energy stores. The phosphorylation potential, which
also depends on the levels of ADP and free phosphate, is more
relevant in this respect [432,169]. Some striking examples of in
vivo ATP depletion in brain, kidney and liver, resulting in
minimal irreversible injury [234], may therefore seem less puzzling. A high correlation between ATP depletion and leakage of
cellular enzymes, over a large range of levels, has also been
considered as proof against a strict relation between enzyme
leakage and cell death [167].

In beating neonatal rat heart cell cultures it was shown that
the extent of anoxia-induced cell death, as measured by cellular
uptake of Trypan Blue, was strictly correlated to released quantities of HBDH [491,7]. In isolated hepatocytes it was also
shown that increased sarcolemmal permeability after anoxia, as
measured by uptake of succinate and Trypan Blue, resulted in
simultaneous leakage of LDH [340].

If it could be shown that some tissue enzymes are eliminated
from the circulation at a rate which could not be compensated by
the quantities of enzyme involved in normal turnover of cells,
the just mentioned question could be simply answered. In that
case some cells which are not replaced, i.e. remain viable,
must also leak enzymes. However, no such examples have been
given. In contrast it seems as if the normal elimination of
circulating tissue enzymes can easily be quantitatively explained
by normal turnover of cells. For instance for LDH, with a normal
plasma concentration of 134 U/l [213], a fractional catabolic
rate constant (FCR) of 0.015 h^{-1} (cf. Chapter 9) and a total
plasma volume of 3 litres, the eliminated quantity per day a-
mounts to 24 x 0.015 x 134 x 3 = 145 U. Normal replacement of
erythrocytes can be approximated by 1% of the total erythrocyte

pool per day, i.e. $0.01 \times 6 \times 5.10^{12}$ erythrocytes per day for a total blood volume of 6 l. The LDH content of erythrocytes is 329 $U/10^{11}$ cells [213], so it follows that loss of LDH amounts to about 1000 U/day. It can be concluded that the loss of LDH from the circulation is only about 15% of the loss of LDH due to normal turnover of erythrocytes.

For a rapidly eliminated enzyme like CK with a FCR of $0.20 \ h^{-1}$ (cf. Chapter 9) and a normal plasma concentration of 28 U/l [538], the total quantity of CK eliminated from the circulation during 70 years in a healthy man with a plasma volume of 3 litres is approximately $70 \times 365 \times 24 \times 0.20 \times 28 \times 3 = 10^6$ U. This amount equals the CK content of 5 kg of skeletal muscle [538]. Considering that skeletal muscle makes up 40-50% of body weight [2] and that skeletal muscle cells have a capacity for regeneration after injury [217], 5 kg of skeletal muscle seems a modest figure for total loss and replacement in a life time. Indeed there are indications for a certain degree of muscle necrosis in normal physiological conditions. Studies in man as well as in various animals demonstrated focal necrosis and loss of enzymes in skeletal and heart muscle after heavy exercise [132,33]. Elevated levels of muscle enzymes in plasma after exercise have frequently been described [411] and explanation of this phenomenon by temporary shifts of enzyme from extravascular compartments to plasma [166] cannot explain continuously increasing plasma enzyme levels in athletes during training [45]. It has also been shown that myocytes are replaced by fibrous tissue in cardiac hypertrophy, resulting in a shift in (iso)enzyme content of the myocardium [377,376].

The results mentioned thusfar cannot prove that living cells may lose enzymes. Still, some results indicate cellular release of proteins under normal conditions or at physiological levels of stress. A number of authors investigated the permeability of cell membranes to plasma proteins under various conditions of stress [501,253,218,389]. The rapidity of cellular uptake of circulating proteins, for instance the uptake of horseradish peroxidase by rat heart cells within 10 minutes of norepinephrine infusion, and also the absence of lasting ultrastructural changes, strongly suggest that this process is still reversible. The same phenomenon was studied in erythrocytes during osmotic lysis. Transient pores in the erythrocyte membrane with diameters up to 1 micrometer were demonstrated, allowing uptake of macromolecules and loss of hemoglobin, followed by resealing of the membrane (cf. [421] for a review). Hemolysis becomes irreversible, however, when the ATP/ADP ratio reaches a critically low level [283]. The occurrence of temporary pores in cellular membranes was already proposed in 1958 in order to explain observations on in vitro incubated rat skeletal muscle [541]. In this study it was noted that the difference in the rates of release of potassium and ALD could be totally explained by the difference in diffusion constants of both substances. The efflux of ALD was thus not selectively inhibited, suggesting a relatively large pore size. Osmotic stress, as used in these studies, could for instance result from increases in cellular osmolarity due to splitting of glycogen, resulting in cellular edema. It has been argued therefore that osmotic stress is a general mechanism operating during energy deprevation [166].

Authors studying dog lymph also tend to consider leakage of enzymes as a normal physiological process [327,461,445]. It was shown, for instance, that enzyme activities in lymph are higher than in plasma while total protein concentration in lymph is lower than in plasma. Moreover, LDH in canine heart lymph has the same isoenzyme pattern as in dog heart while the enzyme content of lymph, as well as lymph flow, increases during heavy exercise. Again these findings leave the point unsettled whether a slight degree of (exertional) necrosis may occur under normal conditions. Also these results contrast with those of a similar study, demonstrating that the ratio LDH/AST in dog heart lymph and in cytoplasmic extracts of dog heart were different in control conditions and became similar after coronary occlusion [297].

Next to the heart, the liver is the most intensively studied organ with respect to quantitative relations between release of cellular enzymes and tissue injury. Unequivocal results are difficult to obtain in this case, since hepatocytes have a much higher capacity to regenerate than myocytes and also because liver injury is often of a chronic nature. In a thorough review of results up to 1968 [411] it was concluded that although some authors have claimed quantitative relationships between release of liver enzymes and tissue damage, most authors feel that hepatocytes may loose moderate quantities of enzyme without being irreversibly damaged. This matter is however still open to discussion. For instance it was found that release of enzymes is a sign of irreversible damage in the rat after administration of toxic agents [177]. In this study, major ultrastructural changes in liver and kidney were found even in cases with moderately elevated plasma levels of LDH and AST.

Some outstanding examples of cell recovery after injury have been presented, as the healing of Purkinje fibres after laser-induced lesions of 100 micrometer in diameter [129], regeneration of Nitella cells after integral removal of the cell membranes [222] or recovery of permeability characteristics in erythrocytes after complete loss of hemoglobin [59]. Obviously some types of cells may release proteins without being lethally damaged.

In spite of discrepancies in the results mentioned above, a recent review [195] concludes that for the beating acutely ischemic or hypoxic heart the onset of significant release of enzymes indicates cell death. For the liver it was also concluded that increased plasma levels of hepatic enzymes, as seen in acute as well as chronic liver disease, are accompanied by cell infiltration and increased fractions of connective tissue in the liver, while exacerbation of enzyme release during chronic liver disease is interpreted as "necrotic attack" [410,414]. It must be concluded that increased loss of enzymes indicates organ damage even although no precise relations are established with histological estimates of the extent of injury. Such precise relations can only be expected if problems as discussed in the preceding section are solved.

Leakage of myocardial enzymes continues for a period of up to 100 hours in patients after acute myocardial infarction (AMI) [527]. This prolonged period of enzyme release strongly suggests a considerable period of extension of tissue injury after the acute event. This is also suggested by the observation that administration of urokinase after AMI considerably shortens the period of release [202], and by the fact that after cardiac surgery there is a much shorter period of leakage of myocardial enzymes than after AMI [203]. The possibility of limiting necrosis after AMI by means of therapeutic interventions, has caused a "borderzone" discussion in the literature [197]. Some authors demonstrated that, after AMI, a relatively large border zone exists between the central necrotic area and normal myocardium [194,151]. This zone could evolve in the course of time and contains potentially salvageable tissue. In a detailed study on CK depletion, however, the quantity of normally perfused tissue in the border zone was defined by accessibility to microspheres of 15 micrometer diameter. Assuming that normally perfused tissue contains normal CK activity, a sharp devision between normal tissue and tissue containing only about 25% of normal CK activity was obtained [206]. Similar results were obtained in a study demonstrating interdigitating normal and ischemic zones, sharply demarcated from each other with respect to glycogen content and electrophysiological behaviour [229]. Comparison of these conflicting results is hampered by the use of different experimental species by different authors and lack of knowledge about transmural, instead of lateral, evolvements. Also, different time-intervals for the assessment of border zones have been used. In the rat it was shown that a zone of reversibly damaged tissue only exists during the first 9 hours after occlusion [151]. This could explain the absence of a border zone as found in the dog 24 hours after occlusion [206]. A marked lack of collateral circulation in the pig, as compared to the dog and man, could explain the absence of a border zone 2 hours after occlusion [229]. The existence of border zones during some time interval after acute coronary occlusion is also indicated by the large number of studies demonstrating the effect of various interventions on experimental infarct size (see [258] for a review).

2.4 Enzyme release from different cellular compartments

As will be discussed in Chapter 4, an important question with
regard to estimation of elimination constants (FCR) and quantification of circulating tissue enzymes is whether such enzymes are
released simultaneously.

For cytoplasmic enzymes of skeletal and heart muscle there is
indeed convincing evidence for simultaneous release. In vitro
incubation of chicken muscle under hypoxic conditions resulted
into parallel release of LDH, CK, MDH, ALD, PGM, and phosphorylase b, ranging in molecular weights from M=70,000 to M=370,000
[119]. Apparently, the increase of membrane permeability occurs
rather sudden because a gradual increase would have resulted in a
delayed release of larger molecules. For in vitro incubated human
and rat heart tissue, simultaneous release was demonstrated for
the enzymes CK (M=80,000), HBDH (M=136,000), AST (M=100,000) and
GPI (M=160,000) [531]. Studies on anoxia-induced release of
enzymes from cultured beating rat heart cells showed a completely
parallel release of CK and HBDH [488] and of HBDH and cytosolic
AST [493].

In perfused rat heart, anoxia as well as reoxygenation resulted in parallel release of MK (M=21,000), CK, AST and GAPDH
(M=144,000) [192]. Hypoxic perfusion of isolated guinea pig
hearts proved that release of a low molecular weight protein as
myoglobin (M=17,600) does not occur earlier than release of CK,
LDH and MDH (M=70,000) [303].

Studies on cardiac lymph after experimental infarction in dogs
and after cardiac surgery in man indicated simultaneous appearance of cytoplasmic (iso)enzymes [327,297,223]. In patients with
AMI, early elevations of plasma levels demonstrated parallel
release of CK and HBDH in quantities proportional to cardiac CK
and HBDH content [527].

In conclusion it is shown in vitro, in isolated muscle and in
vivo, that the change from normal to completely leaky membrane in
the muscle is rapid in comparison to the time in which protein
release takes place. This picture fits into the hypothesis of

loss of intracellular constituents through large pores as discussed in the preceding section.

Different observations have been made in the liver. Isolated
rat liver under moderately hypoxic perfusion shows a correlation
between the rate of enzyme release and molecular weight for
cytoplasmic enzymes [411]. One is tempted to speculate that this
lack of all-or-none response reflects a higher capacity of recovery of hepatocytes - compared to muscle cells - as discussed in
the preceding section. It should also be noted that differences
in cellular rates of release of different enzymes need not be
reflected in differences in overall plasma entrance rates. If the
time scale of evolving tissue injury is long, compared to the
time scale of enzyme release of individual cells, simultaneous
release of different enzymes in plasma will still be observed.

So far, we have discussed only proteins located in the cellular cytoplasma. They diffuse freely to the interstitium as soon
as the cell membrane becomes permeable to macromolecules. The
situation is different for proteins confined to intracellular
compartments or bound to intracellular structures.

The appearance of mitochondrial AST and MDH in plasma after
AMI is delayed considerably compared to the appearance of cytoplasmic enzymes, and indicates severe necrosis [435,223,493,31].
Therefore these enzymes could be excellent markers of myocardial
damage. Unfortunately, the separation of mitochondrial isoenzymes
of AST and MDH from the corresponding cytosolic isoenzymes often
implies inaccuracy due to the separation procedures. In addition,
the quantitative use of mitochondrial enzymes is hampered because
a major part of these enzymes does not appear in the plasma but
remains bound to the mitochondrial matrix and is eventually
inactivated locally [493,435].

The appearance of mitochondrial enzymes in plasma of patients
with liver disease is well documented [410,411,110]. The liberation of mitochondrial enzymes like GLDH, mAST and mMDH from
isolated perfused rat livers is delayed compared to the release
of cytoplasmic enzymes [409,411]. The proportion of mitochondrial
enzyme activity liberated in congestive liver disease is higher
than in hepatitis [411]. The sensitivity of the liver to circu-

latory disturbances was also demonstrated in patients with right-sided heart failure. In those patients, plasma levels of GLDH were 40 times higher than in patients with hepatitis and considerable hepatic necrosis was found at autopsy [180]. Several clinical indices of liver disease are related to the release of mitochondrial enzymes in addition to release of cytosolic enzymes [414,110]. The relative abundance of mitochondrial enzymes leaking from the liver, as compared to enzyme leakage from the heart, may be associated with the observation that liver damage consists of multiple, diffusely located injured sites throughout the liver. Secondly liver damage usually develops relatively slowly compared to AMI. As will be discussed in Section 2.6, diffuse damage may result into decreased local inactivation of enzyme and more complete enzyme release into the circulation than a single localized site of injury. It has also been shown that reperfusion and reoxygenation of ischemic or hypoxic tissue, as could occur during long-lasting circulatory disturbances, result in exacerbation of mitochondrial AST release [493].

The significance of elevated plasma levels of lysosomal enzymes is still a matter of dispute. After the initial observation that ischemia induces a reduction of lysosomal enzyme activity in the particle bound fractions of disrupted hepatic tissue [124], the hypothesis was presented that ischemia-induced acidosis affects the lysosomal integrity with subsequent release of various hydrolytic enzymes into the cytosol of the cell [125]. This process was assumed to initiate the events leading to irreversible cellular damage. Work on in vitro fetal mouse heart, however, showed a retarded release of lysosomal enzymes as compared to the release of cytoplasmic enzymes during anoxia. This is supporting the hypothesis that lysosomes are involved in tissue repair rather than in primary events causing cell death [221]. This second view is substantiated by recent work showing that intracellular diffusion of cathepsin D from the lysosomes into the cytosol does not take place before cell death [122,123].

Lysosomal enzymes like NAG and beta-glucuronidase were found to appear simultaneously with CK in the plasma of patients with

AMI [521]. This study quotes a very low value for the NAG content of human myocardium and it seems that the quantity of NAG appearing in the plasma must be largely of non-myocardial origin and is probably associated with the inflammatory response, secundary to cell death.

As cellular release of enzymes requires major changes in membrane characteristics, it could be expected that release of enzymes bound to the plasma membrane of cells would precede release of cytoplasmic enzymes. Indeed it has been shown that release of membrane-bound LBNA precedes release of CK after anoxia in isolated perfused guinea pig and rabbit hearts [193]. Incubation of liver and kidney tissue in a medium containing proteolytic enzymes caused significant loss of LBNA activity in contrast to activity of AP, an enzyme located in the plasma membrane as well [189]. As indeed no early release of AP from injured tissues has been reported, this supports the hypothesis that early release of membrane markers requires their localization on the outer side of the membrane.

With the exception of a few studies on mitochondrial enzymes and on LBNA, the use of quantitated release of enzymes into plasma has been restricted to cytoplasmic enzymes.

2.5 Pathways for the transport of cellular proteins from tissues to plasma.

Enzymes released from cells are transported to the systemic circulation by means of lymphatic transport and by direct entry into capillaries. As blood flow exceeds lymph flow by several orders of magnitude in most tissues, the lymphatic pathway only dominates in this transport if the entry of enzymes from the interstitium into the capillaries is very slow.

After myocardial injury, enzyme activities in heart lymph are 20-100 times higher than in plasma [327,461,445,297]. However cardiac lymph flow is only 100-150 microlitre/kg/min [445,297] while coronary blood flow is 500-1500 ml/kg/min [4,317] (both values apply to the dog). This implies that although arterio-venous differences in plasma enzyme activity after coronary ligation in dogs [445,455] and after cardiac surgery in patients [174] are small, cardiac enzymes are mainly transported by entry into the capillaries. From quantitative estimates of lymphatic transport of cardiac enzymes after experimental infarction in dogs [445,460] it follows that 15-30% of total enzyme transport takes place via lymph. Lymph drained from the heart is collected in the right lymphatic duct which empties directly in the external jugular vein. Total passage time in lymph is estimated to be about 20 min [445]. In view of the extended period of enzyme release after myocardial infarction this delay is negligible, and it can be concluded that enzymes from the heart are released directly into the plasma.

Capillary permeability in the liver is much higher than in the heart. As will be discussed in more detail in Section 3.2, this implies that proteins released by hepatocytes are transported directly to the plasma. In pathological conditions, impairment of microcirculation due to local edema or necrosis may introduce delays and could alter this situation. This is also true for other organs but the liver may be less susceptible to this complication because diffusely distributed sites of injury, as often occurring in liver, are in close proximity of well-perfused tissue.

Tissues with capillary permeabilities comparable to that in the liver are the spleen, bone marrow, intestinal mucosa and the renal cortex [460,371,166]. It was shown that ^{131}I-labeled albumin injected into the renal cortex of dogs diffused into the bloodstream with a half-life of 10 seconds, while renal ischemia produced an arterio-venous difference in plasma LDH activity after 2 hours of occlusion [459]. Less than 1% of tissue enzymes from renal cortex is transported by renal lymph. In contrast, renal lymph does transport a significant part of ^{131}I-albumin injected into the medulla [460].

Capillaries in skeletal muscle are generally considered as less permeable than those in heart muscle. It has been pointed out, however, that this impression might be caused by the less dense distribution of capillaries in skeletal muscle as compared to that in myocardium [371] (cf. Table 2.2). Most authors agree that tissue enzymes from active skeletal muscle are transported by lymph predominantly. Less than 10% of intramuscularly injected ^{131}I-albumin was released directly into the plasma [460]. As regards the situation in the resting muscle, opinions differ widely. Micro-injected radiolabeled albumin was found to diffuse directly from the interstitium into the bloodstream [460,238], while on the other hand it has been demonstrated that the rise of plasma levels of CK, AST and LDH after ligation of a dog hind limb could be prevented by quantitatively collecting thoracic duct lymph [166].

Capillary permeability of the lung and skin can be compared to that of skeletal muscle. As the capillary surface per unit of tissue weight of the lung is about 50 times higher than of skeletal muscle [371] enzymes are released into the plasma more rapidly.

The appearance of digestive enzymes like amylase and lipase in the plasma after pancreas injury need not be strictly correlated to cellular damage of this organ. These export enzymes are sensitive to obstruction of the pancreatic ducts and may then easily be transported directly into the bloodstream. During its early phase this effect is stimulated by obstruction of local lymphatics and increased capillary permeability. In later stages the lymphatic route of transport becomes the main passage way of digestive enzymes [144,16].

The abdominal, thoracic and pericardial cavities are separated from the circulation by the barrier of the mesothelial membrane. Labeled proteins injected into various compartments in the dog were absorbed most rapidly from the peritoneal cavity (half-life of 6 hours) and most slowly from the pleural cavity (half-life of 23 hours). Protein drainage from these serous cavities occurs predominantly by lymph although the permeability of several surfaces, such as the liver capsule and the diaphragm, is sufficient to allow direct passage of protein into the bloodstream [460].

Table 2.2 <u>Capillary permeability in different tissues</u>

Substance	Molec. weight	Stokes radius (nm)	Heart (S=56)	Skeletal muscle (S=7)	Brain (S=24)
urea	60	0.26	55000(dog) 6600(cat)	7200(man)	3800(dog)
hexose	180	0.36	19000(dog)	3300(man) 2800(cat)	1400(dog)
sucrose	342	0.47	14000(dog)	2200(man) 1500(cat)	180(dog)
inuline	550	1.5	4700(dog)	216(man) 350(cat)	
myoglobin	17000	1.9		216(man) 350(cat)	
albumin	65000	3.6	58(dog)	12(dog) 14(rat)	0.07(man)
IgG	160000	5.6	30(dog)	8(dog)	0.02(man)
$alpha_2$-M	820000	10		4(dog)	0.003(man)

Figures indicate the permeability-surface product PS in ml/kg/h. S is the capillary suface in m^2/kg. Data from refs. [371] and [372] (cf. also Fig 3.1).

Enzymes leaking from brain tissue are effectively prevented from reaching the plasma by highly impermeable capillaries (cf. Table 2.2) and by the blood-liquor barrier. Accordingly, the concentrations of plasma proteins in cerebrospinal fluid are very low and elevations of enzyme levels in cerebrospinal fluid, notably the brain-type isoenzyme of CK, CK(BB), can hardly be correlated to elevations of plasma enzyme levels. This is a serious obstacle in estimating brain damage from plasma enzyme levels [353,74].

Table 2.2 presents data on capillary permeability. These values can be used only as a rough estimation, because capillary

permeability is sensitive to a number of factors that are readily
affected by the applied experimental techniques, e.g. release of
histamine or increased lymph flow. Studies on the transcapillary
escape rate of intravascularly injected labeled albumin in several species resulted into overall values (cf. Chapter 9) which
are 4-6 times lower than would follow from the capillary permeability of skeletal muscle for albumin, when extrapolated to 50%
of body weight.

2.6 Factors preventing tissue enzymes from reaching circulation.

The in-situ activity of intracellular enzymes needs not be
closely related to the activity of enzymes released from the
cell. Changes in physico-chemical conditions between the intracellular and extracellular milieus, for instance differences in
pH, may alter enzymatic activity. Such "sofort"-effects have been
described in the literature [409,411]. Also, many enzymes are
functioning intracellularly in structured environments in which
substrate affinity and catalytic efficiency could differ considerably from those measured in bulk solution.

However, these effects need not complicate the quantitative
relation between tissue damage and released enzyme activity,
because tissue enzyme content is measured in homogenates prepared
in plasma. By homogenisation and sonification the enzymes are
liberated from the cells and their activity can be directly
compared to plasma enzyme activities measured in patients. This
procedure still could introduce discrepancies if the molecular
properties of the enzymes are altered by the release process
itself. In vivo release of cellular enzymes is probably a process
completely differing from liberation of enzymes by homogenisation
and sonification. Different purification procedures for instance
may cause different in vivo catabolism (cf. Section 5.3), although such molecular changes usually do not seem to influence
enzymatic activity. Authors studying this problem have generally
not been able to demonstrate an effect of experimental manipulation of preparations on the values of the Michaelis-constant
(K_m) and maximal turnover rate (v_{max}). This fact supports the

two-state hypothesis of enzyme denaturation, i.e. the assumption that enzyme molecules are either left normally active or are completely inactivated [285].

The effect of autolysis on enzyme activities in necrotic tissue is one of the potential hazards in estimation of tissue damage from plasma enzyme levels. If a significant and variable part of releasable enzyme activity is locally inactivated, tissue damage will be poorly correlated to the quantity of enzyme released into the plasma. For a large number of enzymes in human skeletal muscle, kept at $4^{o}C$ after autopsy, 20-40% of inactivation in 48 hours was demonstrated with the exception of G6PDH which remained stable [408]. Little is known about the comparability of autolytic processes in tissues after death and of events during tissue repair after necrosis in the living organism. Enzyme activities in mouse liver kept in water vapour at $37^{o}C$ are significantly different from the activities in pieces of liver tissue incubated in the abdominal cavity of living mouse [43,44]. Obviously a first step in simulating in vivo necrosis is the introduction of the possibility of protein loss from the necrotic area to the environment.

Several authors investigated in vitro enzyme release from muscle preparations incubated in physiological saline or plasma [166,119,531,541]. Various aspects of in vivo tissue damage can be studied in such preparations as demonstrated by increased release of enzymes from rat and chicken skeletal muscle caused by anoxia, glucose deprivation, high potassium concentrations and by the introduction of metabolic inhibitors like iodoacetate, dinitrophenol and cyanide [541]. It was found that the rate of enzyme release is much more decreased for larger tissue samples, compared to smaller ones, than could be expected for the lower area/volume ratio [119]. The same phenomenon is shown in Fig. 2.1 for anoxic incubated dog heart. From tissue samples of more than 2 grams, less than 10% of LDH, AST and GPI content is released. For samples of human myocardium of about 0.2 g, obtained at cardiac surgery, it was shown that after 100 hours of incubation at $37^{o}C$ total initial LDH(HBDH) and GPI activity was recovered either in the incubation medium or in the residual tissue, while approximately 30% of the total initial CK and AST activity had disappeared [202].

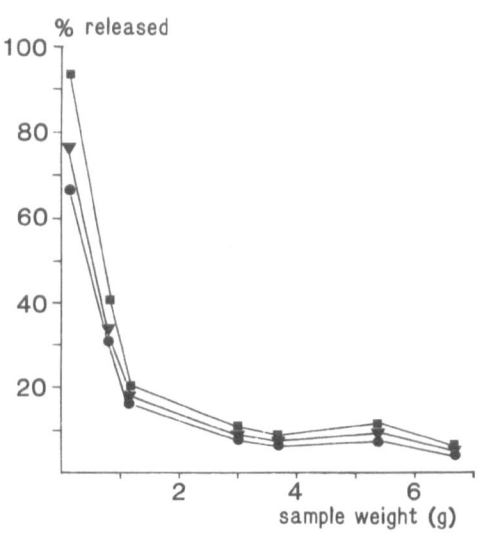

Fig 2.1

Release of CK(▼),LDH(●) and GPI(■) from canine myocardial samples in- cubated in hypoxic dog plasma at 4°C. Total release during 20 hours is expressed as a per- centage of initial enzyme content.

Incomplete recovery of enzymes, as observed in autopsies and during in vitro release from incubated tissue samples, is also observed for CK after experimental infarction in dogs. Comparison of the quantity of CK depleted from the heart with the amount released into the plasma, originally resulted in a recovery of only 30% of depleted CK [424]. This even proved an overestimate, caused by a faulty value for CK distribution space, and was subsequently corrected to 15% [381]. Low in vivo recovery of CK might be attributed to a rapid inactivation of CK in dog lymph. It was shown, for instance, that lymphatic occlusion after expe- rimental infarction in dogs caused a reduction of recovery of CK in the plasma from 19 $\pm$ 2% to 9 $\pm$ 2% (mean $\pm$ SEM, n=6) [94]. This result seems at variance with the relative unimportance of lymph- atic transport of enzymes after experimental infarction in dogs as discussed in the preceding section. An alternative explana- tion, also suggested by the data of Fig. 2.1, is that in a large infarcted area more CK becomes inactivated before escaping into the circulation. This possibility was investigated in a study in which homogeneous experimental infarcts in dogs, obtained by coronary ligation, were compared to scattered infarcts induced by intracoronary injection of microspheres of 0.3 mm diameter [83]. It was found that respectively 18 $\pm$ 3% and 29 $\pm$ 4% (mean $\pm$ SEM, n=9) of CK depleted from the heart was recovered in the plasma. In addition it was demonstrated that in large homogeneous infarcts local inactivation of CK becomes so important that actually less CK is released into the plasma than in smaller homogeneous infarcts [83]. This latter finding may explain earlier observations that a significant correlation between histologically assessed infarct size and total release of CK into the plasma was only found for smaller infarcts, while large infarcts disturbed this correlation because of insufficient release of CK [385]. The recovery of CK in ref. [183] was calculated by equating the elimination constant of CK to the apparent disappearance rate from the plasma (FCR = 0.11 h^{-1} for ligated dogs and FCR = 0.12 h^{-1} for embolized dogs). As will be discussed in Chapter 6, the true elimination constant is underestimated by this procedure. Thus, taking the value of FCR = 0.30 h^{-1} for CK in the dog (cf. Chapter 9), the recovered fraction of CK will be 48 $\pm$ 8% for homogeneous infarcts and 73 $\pm$ 10% for scattered infarctions. The first value is more than 3 times higher than the earlier quoted figure of 15% [381]. Apparently further study is needed in this field.

The phenomenon of in vivo local enzyme inactivation has almost exclusively been studied quantitatively in the heart and for the enzyme CK. Extrapolation to other tissues and other enzymes is precarious. It was shown, for instance, that CK injected into skeletal muscle of dogs was only partially recovered in the plasma, while recovery of AST was complete in the same experiments [504]. It was also shown that CK is rapidly inactivated upon incubation in dog lymph in contrast to LDH [383]. Differences in the stability of enzymes in tissues obtained at autopsy have been discussed in Section 2.2.

2.7 Elimination of tissue enzymes from the circulation.

As will be further discussed in Section 3.4, information on the mechanisms of protein breakdown is surprisingly scarce. Severe hemodynamic disturbances or integral removal of kidneys, liver or spleen hardly affects the rates of elimination from the plasma of a number of enzymes [381,455,142,428,154]. Only for low molecular weight cellular proteins such as amylase, myoglobin and lysozyme that pass the glomerular membrane during plasma filtration, it is known that clearance takes place by urinary excretion when the maximum capacity for reabsorption in the renal tubules is exceeded [184].

Results obtained from a number of studies in the literature seem to indicate independent elimination mechanisms for different enzymes. Plasma elimination rates of CK, as measured after intravenous injection in dogs, were not correlated to elimination rates of AST [506]. This implies that if a certain dog shows for instance relatively rapid elimination of CK, this need not be so for AST. The same applies to the elimination of CK and HBDH in patients after AMI [329]. Mechanisms operating for individual enzyme molecules are also suggested by a large number of studies demonstrating that manipulations of enzyme preparations, such as separation and purification, may induce molecular changes resulting in rapid elimination of specific enzymes (cf. Section 5.3).

The phenomenon of rapid removal from the circulation of damaged enzyme molecules has led to the hypothesis that native enzyme molecules are eliminated after being damaged by proteases in the plasma [356]. This hypothesis was also inspired by observations from the field of intracellular turnover of proteins. It was observed that proteins of high moleculair weight generally showed higher rates of intracellular turnover than proteins of lower molecular weight [127,134]. A larger molecule would have a higher chance of being target for a protease that produces an initial rate-limiting peptide bond cleavage. Indeed, a correlation was demonstrated between the intracellular turnover rate of rat liver enzymes and vulnerability to proteolytic attack [66].

There is little support, however, for this hypothesis when

applied to circulating tissue enzymes. There is no correlation between molecular weight and plasma elimination rates of such enzymes (cf. Chapter 9). Increased values for the Michaelis constant K_m of plasma MDH in a patient with AMI [200], suggestive of a gradual loss of substrate affinity, is probably to be attributed to a varying ratio of cytoplasmic and mitochondrial MDH [435]. After intravenous injections of purified isoenzymes of AST in dogs, no change in K_m could be detected in serial plasma samples [511].

A few studies have considered the disappearance of radiolabeled enzymes. It was found that enzymatic activity and radioactivity disappear simultaneously [381,300,30,407,341]. From this parallel disappearance it was concluded that enzyme elimination takes place by integral removal of enzymatically active molecules from the circulation. A different result, however, was obtained for LDH_5 in the rabbit [358] and for CK(MB) in patients after AMI. The loss of plasma CK(MB) activity in the latter case was much faster than the loss of CK(MB) molecules as measured by an immunological assay [311]. Also it was shown recently that human plasma contains a heat-labile factor that may induce a change in the M-subunit of CK (detectable by electrophoresis) causing a less rapid elimination of CK activity from the plasma [524,88]. This could also explain the observation in the dog, that CK harvested from plasma is catabolized more slowly than CK obtained from heart tissue [440]. These examples illustrate that at least in some cases, inactivated enzyme molecules may remain in circulation for some time, and that molecular alterations may be induced which do not result in immediate removal of molecules from circulation or loss of enzymatic activity (cf. Section 5.3).

Involvement of the mononuclear phagocyte system (MPS; cf. Section 3.4), formerly called the reticulo-endothelial system (RES), in the elimination of circulating tissue enzymes is still a matter of debate. In dogs, intravenous injection of zymosan, a MPS-affecting agent, inhibited the elimination of AST and CK, but not of ALT, from the plasma [511,381]. Infecting mice with Riley virus resulted in higher steady state plasma levels of LDH and GPI with simultaneous functional depression of the MPS as demonstrated by a lower elimination rate of intravascularly injected carbon particles [295]. Another study demonstrated that a number of agents known to stimulate or depress the MPS, correspondingly caused lower or higher levels of LDH and GPI but not of ALT and ALD [294]. The interpretation of these results is however hampered by a few circumstances. Firstly, the MPS seems definitely involved in the elimination of damaged proteins (cf. Section 3.4) and there are many indications that damage may occur in enzyme preparations (cf. Section 5.3). This implies that elimination mechanisms studied with such preparations might not be involved in the elimination of native enzyme molecules. Secondly, it has been stated that administration of MPS-affecting agents may cause a diffuse tissue damage resulting in release of enzymes [12]. This effect could be erroneously interpreted as inhibition of elimination of injected enzymes. Extra release of AST, instead of inhibition of AST catabolism, after administration of zymosan seems indeed apparent from some data in the literature [512]. Whether or not the MPS plays a role in the elimination of native tissue enzymes, the available evidence suggests that this could only apply to rapid elimination [295]. This might indicate that involvement of the MPS in enzyme elimination may become rate-limiting. A possible mechanism for the elimination of tissue enzymes by the MPS could be the formation of complexes of enzyme with IgG, as recently demonstrated for CK [316]. Phagocytosis of protein complexes seems to be a general phenomenon, largely regulated by the size of the aggregates [182].

For the quantification of circulating proteins, the relation must be known between plasma protein concentration and rate of elimination. It is generally assumed that protein elimination from the plasma is a first-order process, i.e. the rate of elimination is proportional to the plasma protein concentration. For the elimination of circulating tissue enzymes, evidence for first-order elimination is indeed convincing. Several studies on various tissue enzymes from the plasma of different species have demonstrated constant values of FCR for a wide range of enzyme concentrations in the plasma (cf. Chapters 6 and 9).

Degradation of enzymes could also occur in the extravascular pool. In this respect a distinction must be made between rapidly and slowly eliminated enzymes. If the rate of elimination is rapid compared to the rate of extravasation, possible extravascular elimination is not important in cases of intravascular input of enzymes. For instance, for GPI a comparison of the elimination rate with the transcapillary escape rate (cf. Chapter 6) shows that only a small percentage of the quantity released into the plasma enters the extravascular space.

If the rate of extravasation cannot be neglected compared to the rate of plasma elimination, direct proof for the absence of extravascular elimination is scarce. This is also true for rapidly eliminated enzymes in those cases where the input of enzyme is not exclusively intravascular. The latter situation occurs for instance for tissue enzymes injected into active skeletal muscle as discussed in Section 2.5. Indeed, such experiments in dogs demonstrated that no extravascular degradation of AST occurred during transport from the gluteus muscle to the bloodstream in contrast to the situation for CK [504].

CHAPTER 3

TURNOVER AND DISTRIBUTION OF PLASMA PROTEINS

3.1 Introduction

The concept of a dynamic state for plasma protein concentrations, in which the steady state concentrations as observed in
plasma reflect the net result of continuous synthesis and breakdown of protein, was developed between 1935 and 1940 [417]. In
the next decade the interest in this field was greatly stimulated
by the introduction of radiolabeled plasma proteins. An impres-
sive number of papers have since been published on the turnover
of plasma proteins. Many of the earlier studies proved to contain
methodological errors, which were only gradually recognized (cf.
Chapters 4 and 5). A selective review of the applied quantitative
methods and the data obtained in plasma protein biology up to
1964, was presented in an authoritative treatise of H.E. Schultze
and J.F. Heremans [417]. Since then, the diversity of specialized
subjects in this field has grown to such an extent that no single
volume compilation covering methods and data could presently be
envisaged.

The present chapter will be strictly limited to those aspects
of plasma protein biology that are relevant to the quantitative
interpretation of (changes in) plasma protein concentrations.
This implies that attention will be paid to the pathways of
protein entrance into the plasma, the distribution of proteins
in the intra- and extravascular compartments and the mechanisms
of protein elimination from circulation.

In several aspects, notably for the exchange of proteins
between different compartments, the behaviour of proteins is much
better known for plasma proteins than for circulating tissue
enzymes as discussed in the preceding chapter. Especially for
albumin much information has become available. For immunoglobulin
G and fibrinogen many studies have been devoted to the deter-

mination of circulatory parameters and also to the changes in these parameters under various pathological conditions. Such changes may cause errors in quantitative estimates of circulating proteins as will be discussed in Chapter 5. The last section of the present chapter therefore contains a summary of data from the literature on the variability of circulatory parameters in man.

3.2 Delivery of plasma proteins to circulation

As will be explained in Chapter 4, a key question in quantification of circulating proteins is whether de novo synthesized plasma proteins pass directly into plasma without previous mixing with extravascular pools. A first step in answering this question is the identification of the sites of synthesis of plasma proteins. By using radiolabeling techniques and organ transplantation, perfused isolated organs, incubated tissue samples, cell cultures and microsomal cell fractions, many authors demonstrated that the bulk of plasma proteins is synthesized either in the liver or in plasma cells [305,417,395,56,391].

As discussed in Section 2.5, identification of the site of synthesis is not sufficient to ascertain the pathway of proteins to circulation. Proteins synthesized in the hepatocytes, for instance, may pass from interstitial fluid to lymph, or they may permeate the capillary wall and enter the bloodstream directly. However, by pulse-labeling with ^{14}C-carbonate and cannulation of the thoracic duct in dogs it was shown that albumin, fibrinogen and haptoglobin pass from the hepatocyte to the plasma directly after synthesis [9,433]. This proves that the hepatic sinusoids are more permeable to macromolecular plasma constituents than any other capillary system. As the sinusoid together with the interstitial fluid draining the hepatocyte can be considered as one mixed pool, the rate of transport of hepatic proteins by lymph and by plasma is determined by the respective flows, which are estimated at 0.0005 ml/g/min for lymph and 0.9 ml/g/min for plasma (dog liver [433]). This means that less than 0.1% of hepatic export proteins is transported by lymph and for quantitative purposes it may be assumed that liver-produced proteins enter directly into the plasma.

It should be mentioned that even if most of the protein transport from organ to plasma takes place by the lymphatic pathway,
models based on intravascular input of protein are not necessarily invalidated. Depending on the localization of the organ and
the speed of lymphatic protein transport, the delay in entering
the plasma may be short enough to render intravascular input a
valid approximation.

Plasma cells are distributed in various tissues, and many of
these cells move continuously back and forth between intra- and
extravascular compartments. As a result, the pathways of protein
entrance into the circulation remain uncertain for proteins
produced by plasma cells. This hampers a quantitative interpretation of changes in plasma immunoglobulin levels in terms of
changes in rate of synthesis. Such complications do not apply to
the interpretation of plasma elimination curves after intravascular injection of radiolabeled immunoglobulins.

Although the main site of synthesis is well established for
most plasma proteins, there is much discussion about additional
sources of protein. Transferrin and alpha$_2$-macroglobulin, for instance, are mainly produced in the liver but may also be produced
by monocytes [443,216]. Another example of a protein with multi-
focal sites of synthesis is clotting factor VIII which is at
least partly synthesized in endothelial cells [228].

3.3 Exchange of protein between plasma and extravascular com-
partments

Estimates of circulating quantities of protein should account
for the effects of extravasation of protein and return of protein
from the interstitium to the bloodstream. It is now generally
accepted that transport of protein between the capillaries and
interstitial fluid may take place by means of three transport
mechanisms, i.e. filtration, diffusion and vesicular transport.
The last type of transport is effected by uptake of protein in
vesicles formed at the membrane of endothelial cells. Vesicles
filled with protein cross the endothelial cells in an apparently

random manner; they may fuse again with the cell membrane and release their protein content in the outside medium.

Diffusional and vesicular transport are assumed to be proportional to a permeability surface factor PS, i.e. the product of a permeability constant P, which is a diffusion constant or a transport rate constant in case of vesicular transport, and the area S of the vascular wall which is permeable to macromolecules. Moreover, these types of transport are assumed to be proportional to the difference in protein concentrations on both sides of the capillary wall:

$$J_D = PS \ (C_p - C_e)$$
(3.1)

where

J_D is the flow of protein (mol/h) due to diffusion or vesicular transport.

PS is the permeability-surface area product (1/h).

C_p is the plasma protein concentration (mol/l).

C_e is the extravascular (interstitial) protein concentration (mol/l).

As discussed before (cf. Table 2.2), values of PS depend on the specific tissue.

Transport of protein by filtration is effected by a bulk flow of plasma through the capillary membrane. This flow is mainly regulated by the hydrostatic pressure difference between capillaries and interstitium and counteracted by the presence of a colloid-osmotic pressure difference. This is generally expressed as [251]:

$$J_v = L_p S (\Delta p - \sum_i \sigma_i \ \Delta \pi_i)$$
(3.2)

where

J_v is the volume flow (1/h)

L_p is the filtration coefficient per unit area (1/N/h)

S is the capillary surface area (m^2)

Δp is the hydrostatic pressure difference (N/m^2) across the capillary wall.

$\Delta\pi_i$ is the osmotic pressure difference (N/m^2) across the capillary wall due to the presence of substance i.

σ_i is the reflection coefficient of substance i that defines the permeability of the capillary wall for this substance. A value σ_i = 1 indicates total impermeability and a value σ_i = 0 indicates that the capillary wall is not a selective barrier for substance i.

Values of σ also depend on the specific tissue considered. For heart capillaries, for instance, typical values are σ = 0.1 for urea (M = 60); σ = 0.3 for sucrose (M = 342) and σ = 0.95 - 1.00 for proteins [372].

The permeability of the capillary wall to proteins is determined by pore size. It is assumed that most pores are small (diameter < 5 nm) and only a few are large (diameter > 20 nm). The presence of pores of different sizes causes a local paracapillary circulation. Through the large pores there is a bulk flow of plasma, mainly regulated by the hydrostatic pressure difference Δp. This flow through the large pores is partially compensated by osmotic adsorption of fluid through the smaller pores and across the endothelial cells. Macromolecules are excluded from the latter pathway. If we consider a single protein and omit the index i, the flow of protein due to filtration may be written as

$$J_f = (1-\sigma)\ J_v\ C \qquad\qquad (3.3)$$

where J_f is the flow of protein (mol/h) due to filtration and C the protein concentration in the volume flow J_v. Due to the local paracapillary circulation, C has a value between the plasma protein concentration C_p and the extravascular protein concentration C_e.

A final transport mechanism of protein to be discussed is the continuous return of protein to the plasma transported by lymph. This flow is equal to $J_l C_l$, where J_l is the flow of lymph (l/h) and C_l is the protein concentration in lymph.

In steady-state condition there is no overall transport of

protein, i.e. $J_D + J_f + J_1C_1 = 0$, or inserting expressions (3.1) and (3.3):

$$PS(C_p-C_e) + (1-\sigma)J_vC + J_1C_1 = 0$$

In the steady-state $J_1 = J_v$. Assuming further that $C_1 = C_e$ and $C = (C_p+C_e)/2$ we arrive at:

$$R = \frac{C_1}{C_p} = \frac{PS + (1-\sigma)J1/2}{PS + (1+\sigma)J1/2} \qquad (3.4)$$

This equation may be derived more rigorously by use of the thermodynamical theory of transport processes [252] and is used in most contemporary studies on transcapillary protein flux data [372,473,379].

Fig. 3.1 shows values of R as measured for plasma proteins and synthetic macromolecules [171,372,337,187]. As shown by the data for the leg, considerable differences were obtained by various authors. It has also been shown that the ratio C_1/C_p is much higher in rest than during physical exercise [337]. The capillary wall is more permeable to synthetic polymers than to proteins of the same molecular weight or with the same Stokes radius [372]. No significant further reduction of permeability is found for molecules with a molecular weight larger than approximately M=60,000.

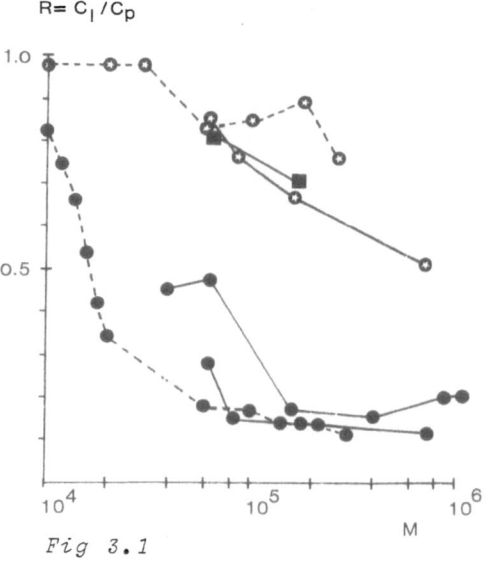

Fig 3.1

Concentration ratio of macromolecules in lymph and plasma. M = molec.mass. Dotted lines indicate synthetic polymers. ●=leg; ○=liver; ■=heart.

This strongly supports the large-pore hypothesis: a certain percentage of the outward flow must pass through pores which are so large that proteins are not selected by their molecular weights [346,171].

In the literature [371,379,473] a variety of expressions have been used to relate the flow through large pores to hydrostatic and osmotic pressure differences and to lymph flow. Different expressions are also used for the relation between C, C_p and C_e. These are in the form C = $(1-\alpha)$ C_p + C_e but the values of α need not be 0.5 as in equation (3.4). Another point of disagreement concerns the existence of differences in protein concentration between interstitial fluid and lymph. A study on nanolitre interstitial fluid samples obtained by micropuncture [400] indeed supports the assumption C_e = C_1 as used in equation (3.4) but investigations based on other techniques indicate that protein concentrations may be higher or lower in lymph than in interstitial fluid [462,461,463,320,71]. Other long-standing points of dispute concern the existence of arterio-venous differences in capillary permeability and the relative importance of diffusion for transport of proteins from the interstitium towards the capillaries.

Several authors have interpreted their data as indicative of considerable arterio-venous gradients in hydrostatic pressure and capillary permeability. The net hydrostatic and osmotic pressure difference is supposed to be directed inward at the venous side. Although this pressure difference is assumed to be small it would results in a considerable inward flow J_v due to a relatively high permeability of the venous capillaries [526]. Other authors, however, assume that J_v is uniformly directed outward [372].

As discussed in Section 2.5, diffusion of proteins from the interstitium towards the capillaries may be found in situations with high interstitial protein concentrations such as found after cellular damage or after intramuscular injection of proteins. It remains to be decided, however, whether this is of importance under normal steady state conditions. In a review of data on albumin concentration in lymph and on total lymph flow in the dog it was concluded that lymphatic return of albumin may fully compensate the total rate of extravasation, thus ruling out any contribution of direct diffusion into capillaries [274]. However, a similar study on a larger number of dogs concludes that as much as 50% of albumin return is effected by diffusion [460]. Such calculations contain uncertainties about the total lymph flow and the albumin content of lymph (cf. Section 2.5). Moreover, the presence of a small rapidly equilibrating extravascular pool, as demonstrated for albumin by several authors [37,464,50], might invalidate these calculations. If in Fig. 3.2, TER_1 is the transcapillary escape rate towards a small compartment V_1 while TER_2 is the usually measured overall transcapillary escape rate of 3-5% of the plasma pool per hour, equality of lymphatic return to TER_2 would mask direct diffusion into the plasma in the magnitude of TER_1. A situation as depicted in Fig. 3.2 might also explain the differences in the ratios between TER and lymphatic return for several proteins, as albumin, IgG and fibrinogen.

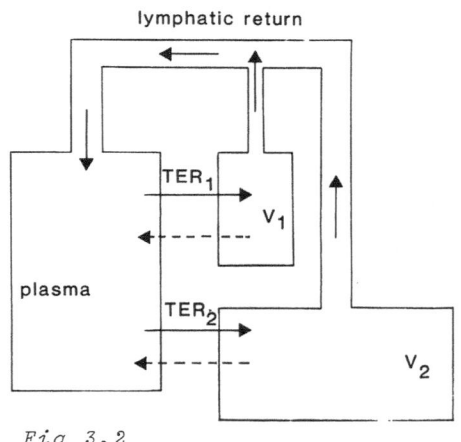

Fig 3.2

Hypothetical 3-compartment model. Broken arrows indicate a possible contribution of diffusion to protein return from the interstitium.

Discrepancies as mentioned can be caused by certain experimental complications. As discussed in Section 2.5, values obtained for permeability-surface area products and lymph flow under experimental conditions may be several times larger than the normal steady-state values of these parameters. Still it is hardly possible to explain the many contradictions and confusions in this field on the basis of complications. The fact that different techniques for the determination of experimental variables result in different values [24] seems to indicate that some of these variables are ill-defined from a physical point of view.

In order to relate extravascular protein concentrations to

values for protein flow and magnitude of extravascular protein pool, the concept of extravascular distribution space is to be introduced. Comparison of the total extravascular quantity of high-molecular dextrans with dextran concentrations in interstitial fluid samples, indicate that extravascular distribution space diminishes with increasing molecular size, but this relation becomes less distinct for molecules larger than M = 50,000 [401]. This effect has been explained [445,526,183] by assuming the presence of a gel phase of mucopolysaccharides in the interstitium from which larger molecules are excluded. Proteins with a molecular weight larger than M = 50,000 are excluded from 30-40% of interstitial fluid volume [401,526]. Molecular sieving, based on smaller distribution volumes for larger molecules, may also explain the relatively rapid extravascular transport of large molecules (cf. Fig. 3.3).

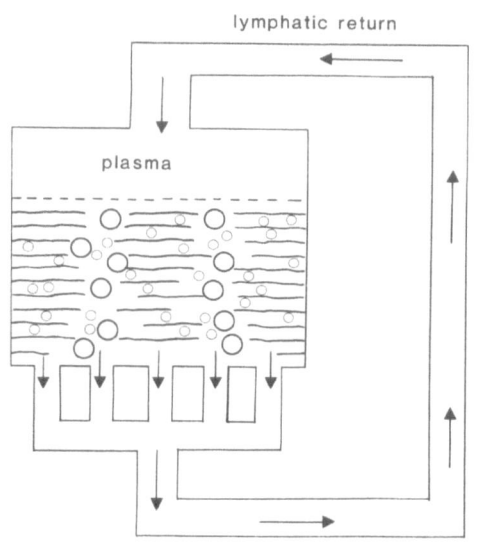

Fig 3.3 *Molecular sieving in the interstitium.*

Values of interstitial fluid volume (IFV) as shown in Table 3.1 and values of C_1/C_p in Fig. 3.1 could be used to estimate the magnitude of the extravascular protein pool. For example, a man of 70 kg has 30 kg of skeletal muscle, 8.4 kg of skin and 9.1 kg of viscera (cf. Table 3.1). Total IFV in muscle and skin is approximately 30x12 + 8.4x500 = 4600 ml and total IFV in viscera 9.1 x 250 = 2300 ml. Taking mean values for

Table 3.1 <u>Interstitial fluid volume (IFV) in various tissues</u>

whole body	skeletal muscle	heart	skin	viscera	species	ref.
(100%)	(43%)	(5%)	(12%)	(13%)		
12-20	8-20		40-60	20-30	man,cat,dog,rabbit	[24]
14	9		50		man	[526]
10					man	[274]
		15			rat	[287]
23	20		40		rat	[248]

Figures indicate IFV in ml per 100 g of wet weight. Figures in parentheses present percentage of total body weight [526,529]. More than 90% of total IFV is located in skeletal muscle, skin and viscera [24].

C_l/C_p = 0.48 for muscle and skin, and 0.60 for viscera (cf. Fig. 3.1), and a value of 3000 ml for plasma volume we find a total extravascular protein pool of (4600/3000)0.48 + (2300/3000)0.60, that is 1.5 times as large as the plasma pool of protein. Correction for extravascular exclusion of protein gives an extravascular protein pool approximately equal to the plasma pool. However, with C_l/C_p = 0.2 (from Fig. 3.1) the values would be approximately halved and definite conclusions cannot be drawn. Studies aimed at directly estimating extravascular protein mass do not produce more consistent results. Authors who determined total tissue albumin by immunological methods reported an extravascular albumin pool of 2.5-3 times the plasma pool [248,249,237]. However, this factor was only 1.6 in another study based on the same technique [111]; this value is in accordance with the values obtained for albumin in metabolic experiments (cf. Chapter 9).

Similar discrepancies are found if the total rate of extra-vasation of albumin is estimated from the data on lymph flow in Table 3.2. Approximately 80% of total lymphatic return in man takes place by way of the thoracic duct [274], and the albumin content of thoracic duct lymph is 75-80% of the plasma albumin content [274,460]. Assuming a plasma volume of 42 ml/kg, this implies that approximately (2.2 x 0.8)/42 = 4% of the plasma albumin pool is returned through the thoracic duct per hour. This value fairly agrees [274] with the overall transcapillary escape rate of 5% per hour as measured after injection of radiolabeled albumin (cf. Chapter 9). However, thoracic duct lymph is not representative of lymph from muscle and skin, which has a considerably lower albumin content (cf. Fig. 3.1). Due to the high lymph flow in liver (cf. Table 3.2) and the high protein content of liver lymph (cf. Section 3.2), as much as 50% of the protein content of thoracic duct lymph may be added by the shunt pathway of the liver [146]; this leads to an overestimate of the lymphatic return of protein from muscle and skin. This can be illustrated by Fig. 3.2 with the liver as rapidly equilibrating compartment. It is concluded that a considerable part of the extravascular return of protein may be effected by direct entry into the capillaries.

Table 3.2   Lymph flow (J_1) in various tissues

Thoracic duct	2.2 (man [274]); 1.3 (dog [187]); 16 (dog [433]; 2.0 (dog [460])
Skeletal muscle	2.5 (man [24]); 0.7-1.3 (man [526])
Heart	0.02(man [72]); 0.1(dog [187]); 6-10(dog [153])
Leg or foot	5.3 (man [24])
Intestine	72 (rabbit [24])
Lung	51 (rabbit [24])
Liver	30 (dog [292])

Figures indicate J_1 in ml per hour per kg of wet weight.

3.4 <u>Elimination of plasma proteins from the circulation</u>

Information on the mechanisms of the breakdown of plasma proteins is surprisingly scarce. For instance for albumin, by far the most studied protein, the mechanism of catabolism is unknown and the site of catabolism is controversial [417,395,391,515]. A major problem proved to be the slow elimination of most plasma proteins. The rate of intracellular degradation of labeled protein fragments far exceeds the rate of protein elimination, and accumulation of label - allowing identification of the site of catabolism - does not occur. A number of glycoproteins that are normally eliminated slowly were shown to be rapidly eliminated after treatment of the protein with neuramidase [23]. This causes hydrolysis of sialic acid residues, leading to exposure of terminal carbohydrate residues which are recognized by specific receptors on hepatocytes. Rapid removal after cleavage of sialic acid residues has been demonstrated for widely different glycoproteins, such as haptoglobin, $alpha_2$-macroglobulin, ceruloplasmin, $alpha_1$-antitrypsin, $alpha_1$-acid glycoprotein, fetuin and clotting factor VIII. Different terminal carbohydrate residues such as galactose, fucose, mannose and N-acetylglucosamine, were found [23,441,499] to serve as recognition markers for hepatic uptake. Moreover, it was suggested that glucosylation of proteins may occur in vivo [121] and that IgG-antigen complexes are removed by the same mechanism after exposure of galactose residues on the IgG-molecule due to formation of the immune complex [477]. This evidence suggests that carbohydrate mediated hepatic uptake might be a general mechanism of protein elimination, but it remains to be established whether in vivo desialization of proteins is physiologically of importance [472]. It must be added that many molecular changes other than desialization may lead to an accelerated elimination of protein, as will be further discussed in Section 5.3.

Damaged protein molecules may be eliminated by the mononuclear phagocyte system (MPS), formerly called the reticulo endothelial system (RES) [497]. The MPS contains fixed "tissue" macrophages and circulating monocytes. Tissue macrophages are widely distributed in the body but most of them are located in the liver (Kupffer cells). To distinguish the uptake of proteins by hepatocytes from uptake by Kupffer cells has been a major problem in studies on protein elimination. One of the main functions of the MPS is clearing the plasma and lymph from particles as micro-organisms and cellular debris. That MPS is involved in clearing heatdenatured protein complexes is indicated by the observation that elimination of carbon particles and of protein complexes shows a mutual inhibition [38,158]. Fluorescine-labeled complexes are mainly accumulated in Kupffer cells [158]. The functional capacity of the MPS in different tissues has been tested by studying the uptake of ^{125}I-labeled heat-aggregated IgG complexes intravenously injected in rats [198]. Ratios of 381:16:12:7:3:1 :0.01 were found for the fractional uptake in respectively liver/ spleen/skin/stomach/large bowel/renal cortex/lung; the fractional uptake was defined as the number of complexes trapped per unit of blood flow measured with labeled microspheres. The fractional uptake of the renal cortex was arbitrarily taken as standard unit. Larger protein complexes appear to be easier trapped by the MPS [182].

For the quantification of circulating plasma protein it must be ascertained whether protein elimination can be considered as a first-order process (cf. Section 2.7). Plasma proteins are indeed generally considered to be eliminated at a rate proportional to the plasma protein concentration. This is mainly indicated by elimination experiments with radiolabeled proteins. In Section 5.2, however, it will be discussed that first-order elimination of the label does not prove first-order elimination of the bulk of protein. In patients and in experimental animals with abnormal plasma protein levels [162,143] it was found that albumin and IgG have a so-called "regulating" behaviour, i.e.fractional catabolic rates are lower or higher for plasma protein levels below or above normal. For haptoglobin and transferrin the opposite has been observed, i.e. fractional catabolic rates are inversely related to plasma protein levels [162]. This behaviour suggests a mechanism of protein elimination that removes a constant quantity of protein per day. True first-order elimination, for a range of 50% to 300% of normal plasma values, was found for fibrinogen and IgM [162,367].

With respect to the question of intra- vs. extravascular e-limination, the situation for plasma proteins is more complicated than for circulating tissue enzymes. Many tissue enzymes are rapidly eliminated and after release into plasma there is insuf-ficient time for a significant extravasation of enzyme. Most plasma proteins, however, are eliminated slowly and a significant fraction of the total protein pool will eventually be located extravascularly, even if the protein enters into plasma directly after synthesis. So the possibility of extravascular elimination of protein becomes an important matter.

Still, there is much evidence for intravascular elimination of plasma proteins. Many authors have noticed that urinary excretion of radioactivity, after injection of radiolabeled protein prepa-rations, is proportional to plasma radioactivity. This is con-vincingly demonstrated by the observation that excretion of radioactivity is delayed after intraperitoneal injection of radiolabeled albumin in patients with ascites [51]. Apparently, plasma proteins are eliminated from the plasma or from a compart-ment "closely connected to" plasma. An exception must be made for immunoglobulins. Extravascular degradation of IgG and IgM has been demonstrated by some authors [8] but was denied by others [15]. Also for other plasma proteins some observations indicate a possible role for extravascular elimination. A study on subcu-taneously injected albumin in patients indicates that 10-20% of the injected quantity was eliminated extravascularly [211]. In experiments with rabbits [211] the fractional catabolic rate constants of ^{131}I-albumin and ^{131}I-fibrinogen were compared to the fractional rates of synthesis of both proteins as measured with ^{14}C-carbonate pulse labeling (cf. Section 4.3). The cata-bolic rate was only 50% of the rate of synthesis during the first few hours after injection and then increased gradually to become equal to the rate of synthesis after approximately 24 hours. This suggests the existence of an extravascular compartment that must be saturated before catabolism can be fully developed.

3.5 Variability of circulatory parameters in man

Calculation of (changes in) circulating quantities of protein from (changes in) plasma protein concentrations requires information about a number of circulatory parameters. This is in the first place the actual value of the plasma volume V_p. In healthy individuals this value can be estimated rather accurately from body weight, using appropriate corrections for age, sex, body surface area etc., but the values of V_p may change in a variety of conditions. Another and often not precisely known parameter is the normal steady state value C_s for the plasma protein concentration in the patient. Plasma protein concentrations may have changed before the first plasma sample is taken and the period of observation is often too short to allow the return of plasma protein levels to C_s. A parameter required for estimating the quantity of protein eliminated from the plasma is the fractional catabolic rate constant FCR. Two additional parameters, the transcapillary escape rate constant TER and the normal steady state value for the ratio of extravascular to intravascular protein pools $(E/P)_s$, are required in order to calculate the extravasated quantity of protein.

As a rule, individual estimates of the values of V_p, C_s, FCR, TER and $(E/P)_s$ are not available, but only mean values as determined for a group of healthy controls or for groups of selected patients. The use of such mean values implies that errors are introduced in proportion to biological variation in parameter values. This problem will be further discussed in Section 5.4. In the present section data from the literature will be discussed on the variability of parameter values for the three best studied proteins in this respect, i.e. for albumin, IgG and fibrinogen, which fortunately cover a wide range of molecular weights.

In addition to true biological variation, data on variability of circulatory parameters also contain a contribution due to experimental error in the estimation procedures. In some cases, such experimental errors may contribute significantly to the total observed variation. As will be discussed in Chapter 4, values of FCR, TER and $(E/P)_s$ as quoted in the literature are usually calculated from the slopes and intercepts of biphasic disappearance curves of proteins from the plasma after an initial intravascular injection of protein. If radiolabeled proteins are used, FCR and $(E/P)_s$ can also be estimated from measurements of excreted radioactivity and the radioactivity retained in the plasma. For the determination of TER, however, measurement of the disappearance curve is indispensable.

As will be discussed in Chapter 4, the value of FCR is mainly determined by the area below the disappearance curve. This area is not much affected by error in protein determination and is rather well defined, provided that the disappearance is followed by a sufficiently long period of time. Calculated values of TER and $(E/P)_s$, however, are less well determined, especially if the value of TER is not much higher than the value of FCR. In that case there is no clear separation between the initial rapid disappearance phase - mainly caused by extravasation of protein - and the subsequent slow disappearance phase. Such ill-defined biphasic disappearance curves may cause large errors of estimation. As shown in Table 3.3 this effect is apparent in variability of values for TER and $(E/P)_s$ for fibrinogen compared to the corresponding values for albumin and IgG. As most authors do not mention the confidence limits of obtained parameter values, it is often difficult to ascertain whether biological variation is significantly overestimated due to such errors.

Table 3.3 also shows that different authors mention different mean parameter values even in healthy individuals, e.g. for FCR of albumin and for $(E/P)_s$ of fibrinogen. Taking into account these systematic differences, it follows that for albumin and fibrinogen the values of FCR and $(E/P)_s$ are not much influenced by various forms of disease. For fibrinogen this aspect will be further discussed in Section 7.5. For albumin exceptions are found in renal failure and after gastrectomy. A lower value of $(E/P)_s$ found in renal failure is probably associated with a considerably expanded plasma volume. The higher value of FCR after gastrectomy probably does not reflect a true increase of metabolic break-down of albumin, but may be caused by gastro-intestinal loss of albumin as found in many gastric disorders

Table 3.3 Variability of circulatory parameters in man.

Protein	Experimental group	Ref.	V_p ±CV*	C_s ± CV	FCR ± CV	TER ± CV	$(E/P)_s$ ±CV
albumin	healthy controls(n=20)	[37]	37±13	45 ± 4	0.0050±14	0.045±31	1.3 ± 15
M=66,500	healthy controls(n=13)	[464]	38± 9	42 ± 4	0.0037±10	0.042±21	1.2 ± 18
	control patients(n=11)	[100]	42±10	45 ±10	0.0043±13	0.067±23	1.4 ± 21
	control patients(n=17)	[231]		39 ±11	0.0039±10		1.5 ± 11
	infections(n=15)	[231]		29 ±16	0.0040±23		1.5 ± 14
	mastectomy(n=7)	[312]	39±24	38 ± 6	0.0040±22		
	renal failure(n=12)	[101]	55±11	30 ±26	0.0033±29		
	hypertensives(n=10)	[347]	40±10	37 ± 5		0.071±14	1.0 ± 37
	gastrectomy(n=7)	[60]		42 ± 7	0.0083±37		
IgG	healthy controls(n=12)	[162]		11 ± 9	0.0023± 7	0.011±11	0.98 ± 11
M=150,000	healthy controls(n=21)	[15]	42±21	13 ±13	0.0026±22	0.016±30	0.92 ± 13
	control patients(n=11)	[99]	38±16	11 ± 7	0.0028±25	0.011±19	0.85 ± 27
	control patients(n=14)	[442]	45± 9	11 ±27	0.0028±18		1.25 ± 14
	plasma cell disease(n=23)	[442]	58±18		0.0032±49		1.34 ± 21
	liver cirrhosis(n=21)	[15]	48±19	31 ±40	0.0036±26		0.72 ± 17
	healthy controls(n=9)	[348]				0.030±23	
	hypertensives(n=7)	[348]				0.047±21	

../2

Table 3.3 (continued)

Protein	Experimental group	Ref.	V_p ±CV*	C_s ± CV	FCR ± CV	TER ± CV	$(E/P)_s$ ±CV
Fibrinogen M=341,000	healthy controls(n=12)	465	36+10	3.6+14	0.010+7	0.023+56	0.19 + 23
	healthy controls(n=35)	482	42+17	2.8+25	0.010+17	0.014+64	0.34 + 38
	mixed patients(n=13)	291	48+31	3.2+41	0.013+15		0.33 + 15
	rheumatoid arthritis(n=11)	466	47+38	3.3+64	0.011+11	0.025+57	0.19 + 21
	glomerulonephritis(n=10)	467	37+22	6.2+28	0.010+16	0.029+33	0.17 + 29
	haemophilia(n=12)	468	42+21	3.5+26	0.015+10	0.033+25	0.22 + 41
	liver cirrhosis(n=50)	482	47+21	2.5+41	0.034+37	0.020±37	0.32 + 37
	liver carcinoma(n=5)	291	46+11	4.8+11	0.015+6		0.30 + 10

*V_p = mean plasma volume in ml per kg of body weight; C_s = mean steady state plasma concentration of protein in gram per litre of plasma; FCR = mean fractional catabolic rate constant i.e. the fraction of the plasma protein pool eliminated per hour; TER = mean transcapillary escape rate constant i.e. the fraction of the plasma protein pool extravasated per hour. In studies using more than two compartments, TER represents the total rate constant of protein extravasation. $(E/P)_s$ = mean steady state ratio of extravascular to intravascular quantities of protein; CV = coefficient of variation i.e. standard deviation expressed as a percentage of the mean.

[394]. The same is observed in nephrosis due to proteinuria. Increased values of $(E/S)_p$ are found in various forms of oedema. In myxoedema this is accompanied by a decreased fractional catabolic rate of albumin [278,396]. Low plasma albumin concentrations, as found in malnutrition, severe liver injury or in persons living in a hot climate, also result in decreased values of FCR [394]. This reflects a departure of first-order elimination of albumin as discussed in the preceding section. However, this effect is insufficiently pronounced to be observed in cases with moderately lower plasma albumin concentrations.

Variability of TER, as shown in Table 3.3, exceeds the variability of the other parameters. Higher values of TER in hypertension reflect the increased capillary filtration pressure in such patients [347,348]. The "large pore" aspect of transcapillary transport of macromolecules, as discussed in Section 3.3, is reflected by the absence of significantly different values of TER for IgG (M = 150,000) and fibrinogen (M = 341,000).

Little is known about the variability in time of circulatory parameters in one and the same individual. The long period of observation needed for obtaining data as presented in here are prohibitive in repeating measurements in the individual patient. A few studies in which such measurements were done [37,312,178] seem to indicate a trend of lower variability in individual patients than between individuals. However, the data are scarce and exceptions to the general trend can be found. An example of a well-documented change of V_p in time in patients after acute myocardial infarction will be discussed in Chapter 7.

CHAPTER 4

METHODS AND MODELS USED IN QUANTITATIVE STUDIES

OF CIRCULATING PROTEINS

4.1 Introduction

Circulatory systems as studied in this chapter consist of an intravascular (plasma) compartment which may be connected to some extravascular compartments. Each compartment contains a well-mixed pool of protein. It is assumed that the system is originally in steady-state conditions while at time t=0 some process starts resulting in intravascular release of protein. This input process may vary from a single injection of a bolus of radio-labeled protein to a long-lasting change in the rate of synthesis of the protein considered. Due to the input of protein, the plasma protein pool $P(t)$ and the extravascular protein pool(s) $E_i(t)$, $i = 1,2...n$ will change in time. The main problem studied in this chapter is to calculate cumulative release of protein into the plasma, between t=0 and time t, from the changes in $P(t)$ measured in the course of time.

A large number of different circulatory models have been used in the literature for quantitative interpretation of changes in plasma protein concentrations. A crucial assumption which is almost universally - although mostly implicitly - made is that one is dealing with a linear compartmental system. Such a system is usually defined by the requirement that the transfer of protein from a compartment to any other part of the system is proportional to the quantity of protein present in the compartment, with transfer constants which remain constant during the period of observation. Alternatively the linearity of the system can be defined by the property that the response of the system to a series of protein inputs can be simply obtained by adding the responses to the individual inputs. This latter definition implies that a linear system can be defined by the response to a single input of protein. If such a response can be characterized by a mathematical expression, no further information on the details of the circulatory system is required for quantification of an arbitrary release of protein.

However, most studies on circulating proteins are focussed on collecting specific physiological data such as the transcapillary exchange rate or the value of the fractional catabolic rate constant. In these studies, the mathematical expression for the response of the system to a single input of protein is only of interest if it can be explained by underlying physiological models and mechanisms. A proliferation of different models have been presented in the literature, which are mathematically equivalent and can be reduced to a few basically different physiological models, presented in Section 4.2. Only those models are discussed which have been applied to circulating proteins. More complicated models, including non-linear ones, have been used in other fields of biology and medicine [230, 77]. Section 4.2 is concluded by considering information which can be obtained without specific assumptions about the number and arrangement of the extravascular compartments.

A survey of different models and methods for the determination of model parameter values, as used by different authors, is given in Section 4.3. The models are translated in the basic model representations introduced in Section 4.2.

It is often possible to study changes in plasma protein concentrations due to various forms of disease. Leakage of tissue enzymes from damaged organs or transient increases in the rate of synthesis of acute phase proteins after trauma, are examples of naturally occurring inputs of protein. Such inputs can, in principle, be used for the characterization of the response of the circulatory system, instead of injections of protein. In Section 4.4 it is shown, however, that it is inherently impossible to obtain circulatory parameter values from naturally occurring inputs of a single protein. This limitation can be overcome if two different proteins are released simultaneously into the plasma. In that case, circulatory parameters may be obtained.

4.2 Basic compartmental models

One-compartment model

Elimination of proteins injected into plasma can often be described by exponential disappearance curves. If one unit of protein is injected intravascularly at time t=0, a simple mono-exponential disappearance is sometimes observed:

$$C_p(t) = C_o e^{-kt} \tag{4.1}$$

where $C_p(t)$ is the plasma protein concentration in units of protein per litre of plasma at time t, and k and C_o are constants obtained by fitting the experimental disappearance curve to the expression (4.1). Equation (4.1) implies that in the normal steady state, i.e. prior to t=0 and after an infinitely long time interval (t → ∞), no protein is present in the plasma. If this is not true and we have a normal steady-state protein concentration C_s, this value must be subtracted from the measured plasma protein concentrations in order to obtain equation (4.1).

If one considers a series of intravascular inputs of F_i units of protein given at times t_i, i=1,2,3...n, the linearity of the system implies that the resulting plasma protein concentration can simply be written as the sum of functions:

$$C_p(t) = \sum_{i=1}^{n} F_i C_o e^{-k(t-t_i)}$$

or for a continuous time-dependent input of F(t) units per hour:

$$C_p(t) = \int_o^t F(\tau) C_o e^{-k(t-\tau)} d\tau = C_o e^{-kt} \int_o^t F(\tau) e^{k\tau} d\tau \tag{4.2}$$

In order to find the quantity of protein entering the plasma from t=0 up to time t, the quantity $A(t) = \int_o^t F(t)dt$ must be calculated. Differentiating equation (4.2) one obtains:

$$\frac{d}{dt} C_p(t) = -k \, C_p(t) + C_o \, F(t)$$

or after rearranging of terms and integration

$$A(t) = \int_o^t F(\tau)d\tau = \frac{1}{C_o} [C_p(t) + k \int_o^t C_p(\tau)d\tau] . \qquad (4.3)$$

This example shows that by studying the effect of a bolus injection of protein, i.e. by determination of the parameters C_o and k from the disappearance curve (4.1), we have characterized the system. Knowing these parameters, for instance by measurement of the intercept with the y-axis and the slope of the straight line obtained from a semi-logarithmic plot of (4.1), any input of protein can be calculated by use of equation (4.3). This result is obtained without any reference to a specific circulatory model or physiological mechanism.

Let us now consider the model given in Fig. 4.1. The plasma is considered as a well-mixed single compartment with volume V_p and protein concentration $C_p(t)$. The total plasma protein pool at time t is denoted by P(t). The protein is eliminated from the plasma by a first-order catabolic mechanism, i.e. the rate of elimination is given by:

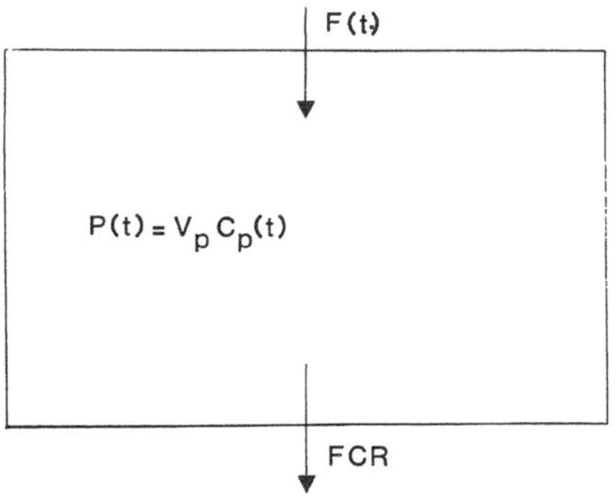

$$P(t) = V_p \, C_p(t)$$

$$\frac{d}{dt} P(t) = - FCR . P(t)$$

Fig 4.1 One-compartment model.

where FCR is the fractional catabolic rate constant.

Solving this equation for an intravascular bolus injection of one unit of protein, given at t=0, one obtains:

$$P(t) = P_o \, e^{-FCR \cdot t} \text{ with } P_o = 1, \text{ or } C_p(t) = \frac{1}{V_p} e^{-FCR \cdot t}.$$

Using the model of Fig. 4.1, we now have explained the response curve (4.1) and the constants C_o and k have a physiological
significance: C_o is the reciprocal plasma volume and k is the
fractional catabolic rate constant. Equation (4.3) can now be
written as

$$A(t) = P(t) + FCR. \int_o^t P(\tau)d\tau \qquad (4.4)$$

and this equation is self-evident: the total quantity of protein
released into plasma consists of the protein still present in the
plasma, P(t), and the quantity of protein which has been eliminated up to time t, i.e. $FCR. \int_o^t P(\tau)d\tau$.

In this example, the specific advantages of the two different
approaches are apparent. The "mathematical" approach is straight-
forward and practical. The problem of quantification is solved as
soon as we have a mathematical expression which fits the response
curve obtained from a bolus injection of protein. The "physiological" approach is more complicated because the response curve
has to be explained by an appropriate model. However, this approach has the advantage that physiological interpretation of
parameters allows independent checks of parameter values. The
value of V_p in Fig. 4.1 could for instance be checked by dilution
of radiolabeled albumin. This example also shows that physiological interpretation can make some results self-evident which require elaborate calculations and remain rather abstract in the
mathematical approach.

Two-compartment model

Proteins injected into plasma often do not disappear mono-
exponentially but show an initial rapid disappearance followed by
a slower elimination phase. Such biphasic curves are observed in
the majority of studies on the turnover and distribution of
plasma proteins. If the response curve to an intravascular bolus
injection of protein can be described by a sum of two exponential
curves, the total release of protein into plasma between t=0 and
time t, A(t), can again be simply calculated by use of the expression presented in Table 4.1.

Such a biphasic response curve can be explained by the two-compartment model presented in Fig.4.2. Proteins no longer remain confined to the plasma pool P(t) but may enter an extravascular protein pool E(t). The rate of extravasation of protein, i.e. the rate of transport from P(t) to E(t), is given by TER.P(t) where TER is the fractional transcapillary escape rate constant. Proteins are transported back from E(t) to P(t) at a rate ERR.E(t) where ERR

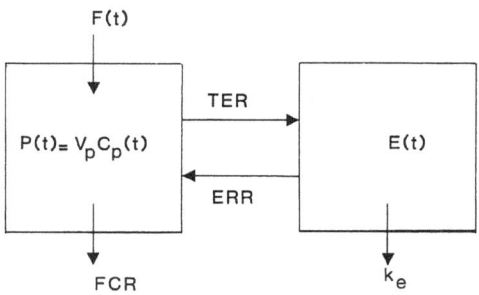

Fig 4.2   General two-compartment model with intravascular input of protein.

is the fractional extravascular return rate constant. Apart from intravascular catabolic breakdown of protein at a rate FCR.P(t), proteins may also be eliminated extravascularly at a rate k_e.E(t) where k_e is the fractional extravascular elimination rate constant. From Fig. 4.2 we find that in a steady state, i.e. $\frac{d}{dt}$ E(t)=0, we must have:

$$TER.P_s = (ERR+k_e).E_s, \text{ or } (E/P)_s = TER/(ERR+k_e).$$

It should be realized that only for certain ranges of parameter values, additional circulatory compartments will result in additional observable exponential disappearance phases. If the value of TER in Fig. 4.2 would for instance be very small compared to FCR, no biphasic disappearance would occur and the protein would be simply eliminated from the plasma before E(t) could be build up. For very large values of TER and ERR, P(t) and E(t) form one single well-mixed distribution space and again a simple monophasic disappearance would be observed. These examples illustrate that the body could contain very slowly exchanging pools which cannot be discovered by studying the response to intravascular bolus injection of protein.

It can be shown (cf. Appendix) that the response to an intra-vascular bolus injection of one unit of protein in this model is given by:

$$P_b(t) = P_1 e^{-k_1 t} + P_2 e^{-k_2 t} \quad \text{with} \quad P_1 + P_2 = 1$$

$$E_b(t) = R_1 e^{-k_1 t} + R_2 e^{-k_2 t} \quad \text{with} \quad R_1 + R_2 = 0$$

(4.5)

with P_1, P_2, k_1, $k_2 > 0$.

The parameters P_1, P_2, R_1, R_2, k_1 and k_2 depend upon the model parameters in Fig. 4.2 according to:

$$k_{1,2} = \tfrac{1}{2}(H_1 \pm \sqrt{H_1^2 - 4H_2}) \qquad H_1 = FCR + TER + ERR + k_e \qquad (4.6)$$
$$H_2 = FCR.ERR + FCR.k_e + TER.k_e$$

$$P_1 = (ERR + k_e - k_1)/(k_2 - k_1) \; ; \; P_2 = 1 - P_1$$
$$R_1 = TER/(k_2 - k_1) \; ; \; R_2 = -R_1.$$

The model parameters in Fig. 4.2 can be calculated from the response curves (4.5) by use of the equations (cf. Appendix):

$$TER = R_1(k_2 - k_1)$$
$$ERR + k_e = P_1 k_2 + P_2 k_1$$
$$TER.ERR/(ERR + k_e) = P_1 P_2 (k_2 - k_1)^2 / (P_1 k_2 + P_2 k_1)$$
$$FCR + k_e.TER/(ERR + k_e) = k_1 k_2 / (P_1 k_2 + P_2 k_1).$$

(4.7)

In many applications of this model, $E_b(t)$ cannot be measured separately after an intravascular bolus injection of protein. This implies that the first equation (4.7) cannot be used because R_1 is unknown. The remaining three equations (4.7) do not allow unequivocal determination of all four model parameters TER, ERR, k_e and FCR, and we have in fact a family of equivalent models which cannot be discriminated. In that case, an additional assumption is required in order to allow physiological interpretation of parameter values. Most frequently it is assumed that no extravascular elimination of protein occurs, i.e. $k_e = 0$. As discussed in the preceding chapters, this assumption has been directly validated for a number of proteins.

In the absence of extravascular elimination of protein it follows from equation (4.7) that the model parameters can be calculated from the plasma disappearance curve $P_b(t)$ by use of the relations:

$$ERR = P_1 k_2 + P_2 k_1$$

$$TER = P_1 P_2 (k_2 - k_1)^2 / (P_1 k_2 + P_2 k_1) \qquad (4.8)$$

$$FCR = k_1 k_2 / (P_1 k_2 + P_2 k_1).$$

Comparison of (4.7) and (4.8) shows that we have the following correspondencies, where the parameters of the model without extravascular elimination of protein are denoted by accents:

$$k_e' = 0$$
$$ERR' = ERR + k_e$$
$$TER' = TER.ERR/(ERR + k_e) \qquad (4.9)$$
$$FCR' = FCR + k_e.TER/(ERR + k_e).$$

Equation (4.9) implies that if it is erroneously assumed that no extravascular elimination of protein occurs, the fractional catabolic rate constant FCR and the extravascular return rate constant ERR are overestimated while the transcapillary escape rate constant TER is underestimated. This also implies that the extravascular protein pool is underestimated because we have:
$(E'/P')_s = TER'/ERR' = TER.ERR/(ERR + k_e)^2 < TER/(ERR + k_e) = (E/P)_s.$

For a two-compartment model without extravascular elimination of protein and parameter values FCR', TER' and ERR' ($k_e' = 0$), the extravascular compartment can be regarded as a single compartment with input function TER.P(t) and elimination constant ERR'. In analogy to equation (4.2) one may then write:

$$E(t) = TER' \int_0^t P(\tau) \, e^{-ERR'(t-\tau)} \, d\tau.$$

Table 4.1   Quantification of protein release into plasma from the response to an intravascular bolus injection.

Monophasic response: $P_b(t) = P_0 e^{-kt}$ $(P_0 = 1)$

$$P(t) = P_0 \int_0^t F(\tau) e^{-k(t-\tau)} d\tau$$

$$A(t) = P(t) + k \cdot \int_0^t P(\tau) d\tau$$

Biphasic response: $P_b(t) = P_1 e^{-k_1 t} + P_2 e^{-k_2 t}$ $(P_1 + P_2 = 1)$

$$P(t) = \sum_{i=1}^2 P_i \int_0^t F(\tau) e^{-k_i(t-\tau)} d\tau$$

$$A(t) = P(t) + A_0 \int_0^t P(\tau) d\tau + A_1 \int_0^t P(\tau) e^{-a(t-\tau)} d\tau$$

$a = P_1 k_2 + P_2 k_1$; $A_0 = k_1 k_2/a$; $A_1 = -(k_1-a)(k_2-a)/a$

Triphasic response: $P_b(t) = P_1 e^{-k_1 t} + P_2 e^{-k_2 t} + P_3 e^{-k_3 t}$ $(P_1 + P_2 + P_3 = 1)$

$$P(t) = \sum_{i=1}^3 P_i \int_0^t F(\tau) e^{-k_i(t-\tau)} d\tau$$

$$A(t) = P(t) + A_0 \int_0^t P(\tau) d\tau + A_1 \int_0^t P(\tau) e^{-a(t-\tau)} d\tau + A_2 \int_0^t P(\tau) e^{-b(t-\tau)} d\tau$$

$a,b = \frac{1}{2}(H_1 \pm \sqrt{H_1^2 - 4H_2})$; $H_1 = P_1(k_2+k_3) + P_2(k_1+k_3) + P_3(k_1+k_2)$

$$H_2 = P_1 k_2 k_3 + P_2 k_1 k_3 + P_3 k_1 k_2$$

$A_0 = \dfrac{k_1 k_2 k_3}{ab}$; $A_1 = \dfrac{(k_1-a)(k_2-a)(k_3-a)}{a(a-b)}$; $A_2 = \dfrac{(k_1-b)(k_2-b)(k_3-b)}{b(b-a)}$

$P_b(t)$: plasma pool after i.v. bolus injection of one unit.
$P(t)$: plasma pool during i.v. release of $F(t)$ units per hour.
$A(t)$: cumulative i.v. release up to time $t (= {_0\int^t} F(\tau) d\tau)$.

The total intravascular release A(t) may in that case be written as:

$$A(t) = P(t) + TER' \int_0^t P(\tau) \, e^{-ERR'(t-\tau)} \, d\tau + FCR' \int_0^t P(\tau) d\tau. \quad (4.10)$$

Substitution of (4.9) into this equation results in the following equation for the general two-compartment model:

$$A(t) = P(t) + [ERR/(ERR+k_e)]E(t) + [FCR+k_e \cdot TER/(ERR+k_e)] \int_0^t P(\tau) d\tau$$

$$\text{with } E(t) = TER \int_0^t P(\tau) \, e^{-(ERR+k_e)(t-\tau)} \, d\tau. \quad (4.11)$$

Substitution of (4.8) into (4.11) shows that the latter equation is equivalent to the expression for A(t) in case of a biphasic response $P_b(t)$ as presented in Table 4.1.

Three-compartment models

The situation of a triphasic response to an intravascular bolus injection of protein is also met in practice. A model which could explain such a response is presented in Fig. 4.3.

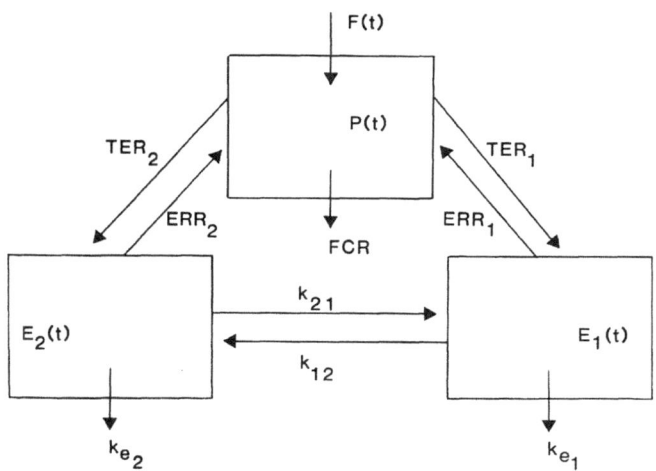

Fig 4.3 General three-compartment model with intravascular input of protein.

For this model the response to an intravascular bolus injection
of one unit of protein can be written as:

$$P_b(t) = P_1 e^{-k_1 t} + P_2 e^{-k_2 t} + P_3 e^{-k_3 t}; \quad P_1 + P_2 + P_3 = 1$$
$$E_{1b}(t) = R_1 e^{-k_1 t} + R_2 e^{-k_2 t} + R_3 e^{-k_3 t}; \quad R_1 + R_2 + R_3 = 0 \quad (4.12)$$
$$E_{2b}(t) = S_1 e^{-k_1 t} + S_2 e^{-k_2 t} + S_3 e^{-k_3 t}; \quad S_1 + S_2 + S_3 = 0$$

In practical applications of this model, one is again limited by
the fact that, $E_{1b}(t)$ and $E_{2b}(t)$ cannot be measured separately.
At best one may estimate $E_{1b}(t) + E_{2b}(t)$ and often only $P_b(t)$ can
be accurately determined. In that case only 5 independent parameters can be estimated from the response curve. As the model in
Fig. 4.3 contains 9 independent parameters, a significant simplification of this model is required in order to obtain parameters
that can be experimentally determined. The reduction most frequently made, is to consider a so-called mammillary system, i.e.
a system in which the input of protein occurs in a central compartment interacting with all other compartments, without extravascular elimination of protein and without direct interaction
between extravascular compartments. Such a model is presented in
Fig. 4.4.

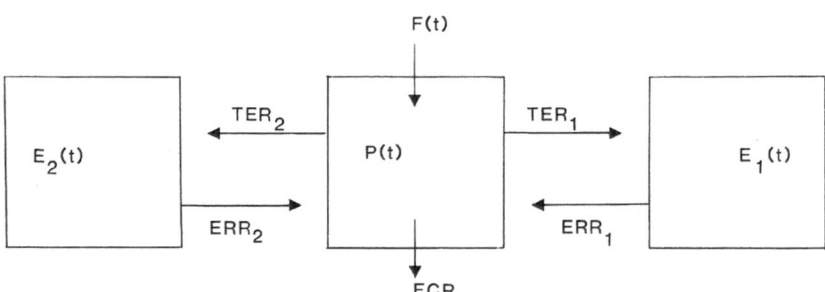

*Fig 4.4   Three-compartment mammillary system as used by
Matthews, ref.301.*

An intravascular bolus injection of one unit of protein into a
mammillary system again results in the triphasic response curves
(4.12) while the parameters in the plasma curve P(t) can be

expressed in the model parameters of Fig. 4.4 according to (cf. Appendix):

$$P_1 = \frac{(ERR_1-k_1)(ERR_2-k_2)}{(k_2-k_1)(k_3-k_1)} \; ; \; P_2 = -\frac{(ERR_1-k_2)(ERR_2-k_2)}{(k_1-k_2)(k_3-k_2)} \; ; \; P_3 = 1-P_1-P_2$$

where the exponential constants k_1, k_2 and k_3 are the roots of the cubic expression (cf. Appendix):

$$k^3 + H_2 k^2 + H_1 k + H_0 = 0$$

(4.13)

with

$H_2 = FCR + TER_1 + TER_2 + ERR_1 + ERR_2$

$H_1 = FCR.ERR_1 + FCR.ERR_2 + TER_1.ERR_2 + TER_2.ERR_1 + ERR_1.ERR_2$

$H_0 = FCR.ERR_1.ERR_2$

It can be shown that for the mammillary system presented in Fig. 4.4, the coefficients P_1, P_2 and P_3 must be positive. The exponential constants k_1, k_2 and k_3 also have positive and real values.

Reversely, one may express the model parameters of the mammillary system in the parameters obtained from the response curve by use of the equations (cf. Appendix):

$ERR_{1,2} = \frac{1}{2}(H_1 \pm \sqrt{H_1^2 - 4H_2})$ with $H_1 = P_1(k_2+k_3)+P_2(k_1+k_3)+P_3(k_1+k_2)$

$H_2 = P_1 k_2 k_3 + P_2 k_1 k_3 + P_3 k_1 k_2$

$$TER_{1,2} = \pm \frac{(k_1-ERR_{1,2})(k_2-ERR_{1,2})(k_3-ERR_{1,2})}{(ERR_{1,2}-ERR_2)ERR_{1,2}}$$

(4.14)

$FCR = 1/(P_1/k_1 + P_2/k_2 + P_3/k_3)$

If this analysis is applied to a three-compartment mammillary system in which extravascular elimination of protein does occur, i.e. $k_{e1} \neq 0$ and/or $k_{e2} \neq 0$, we have the following correspondencies:

$$k_{e1}' = k_{e2}' = 0$$
$$FCR' = FCR + k_{e1} \cdot TER_1/(ERR_1 + k_{e1}) + k_{e2} \cdot TER_2/(ERR_2 + k_{e2})$$
$$ERR_1' = ERR_1 + k_{e1}$$
$$ERR_2' = ERR_2 + k_{e2} \qquad\qquad (4.15)$$
$$TER_1' = TER_1 \cdot ERR_1/(ERR_1 + k_{e1})$$
$$TER_2' = TER_2 \cdot ERR_2/(ERR_2 + k_{e2})$$

Again we find that extravascular elimination, if not properly appreciated, results in overestimation of the fractional catabolic rate constant and extravascular return rate constants, while the transcapillary escape rates are underestimated.

In analogy with the two-compartment model we find for the total intravascular input in the model of Fig. 4.4:

$$A(t) = P(t) + E_1(t) + E_2(t) + FCR \cdot \int_o^t P(\tau)d\tau \qquad \text{or}$$

$$A(t) = P(t) + TER_1\int_o^t P(\tau)e^{-ERR_1(t-\tau)}d\tau + TER_2\int_o^t P(\tau)e^{-ERR_2(t-\tau)}d\tau$$

$$+ FCR\int_o^t P(\tau)d\tau. \qquad\qquad (4.16)$$

Substitution of equation (4.14) into this equation again shows that (4.16) is identical to the expression for A(t) in case of a triphasic response in Table 4.1.

A three-compartment model which is not equivalent to the mammillary model is shown in Fig. 4.5. An intravascular bolus injection of one unit of protein again results in the triphasic response curves (4.12) but, in contrast to the situation for the mammillary system, at least one of the coefficients P_1, P_2 or P_3 must have a negative value. This implies that triphasic plasma curves $P_b(t)$ with positive values of P_1, P_2 and P_3 are inconsistent with the model presented in Fig. 4.5, and such curves were actually found in ref. [154]. The exponents k_1, k_2 and k_3 may now have complex values, i.e. the response curves $P_b(t)$ may show damped oscillations.

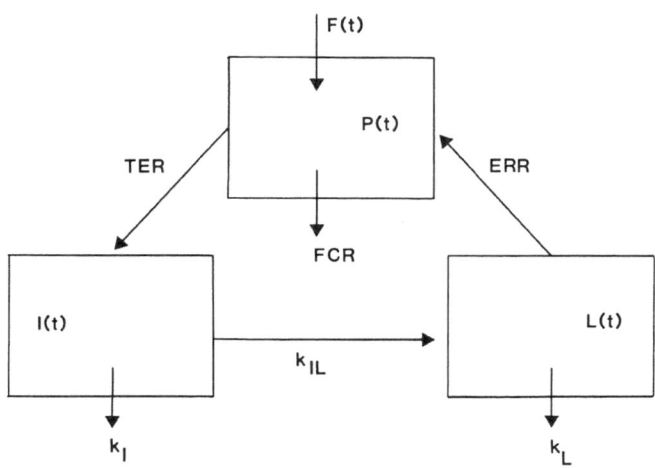

*Fig 4.5   Three-compartment model with interstitial pool I(t)
and lymph pool L(t), as used by Fleisher, ref.154.*

General multi-compartment models

From the preceding it is apparent that a system with n exchanging compartments will generally show a n-exponential plasma
disappearance curve $P_b(t)$. A non-exchanging pool, however, will
not result in an additional exponential. This is illustrated in
Fig. 4.6 where a six-compartment model is presented as used for
the interpretation of data on the turnover and distribution of
radiolabeled albumin. This model is essentially the general
three-compartment model from Fig 4.3, but some non-exchanging
pools have been added. It was noted that there is a time delay
between the disappearance of radiolabel from the plasma pool P(t)
and the appearance of radioactivity in the urinary excretion pool
U(t). So a "buffer" pool $E_3(t)$ of radioactive protein degradation
products was added. It was also noted that total excreted activity did not approach 100% of total injected activity. So an extravascular compartment $E_4(t)$ of radioactive protein degradation

products was added, which acts as a "body sink", i.e. protein entering this compartment is not returned to the circulation. Other authors, however, reported complete excretion of injected radioactivity [37].

Apart from changing the values of elimination constants, the addition of non-exchanging pools in Fig. 4.6 has no effect on the disappearance curves $P_b(t)$, $E_{1b}(t)$ and $E_{2b}(t)$ after intravascular bolus injection. It is irrelevant for protein kinetics whether proteins are simply removed, as in Fig. 4.3, or transported to the urine and to a body sink, as in Fig. 4.6. So again triphasic curves will be observed.

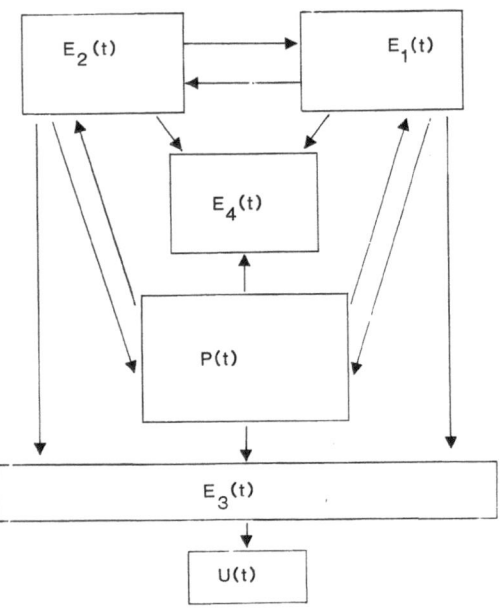

Fig 4.6   A six-compartment
model as used by
Lewallen, ref. 277.

Models as presented in Fig. 4.6 raise the problem of identification of model parameters. For a model with n compartments, each compartment may introduce n model parameters, i.e. n-1 rate constants for the transfer to other compartments and one elimination constant. This implies that such a model may contain n^2 independent model parameters. The quantity of information which can be extracted from the plasma disappearance curve $P_b(t)$ is rather limited. Due to experimental scatter in data points $P_b(t)$ usually cannot be resolved in more than three exponentials from which five independent parameters are obtained: k_1, k_2, k_3, P_1 and P_2 (cf. 4.12). Measurement of an additional compartment, for instance the urinary excretion $U(t)$, in this case only adds two extra parameters because the exponential constants k_1, k_2 and k_3 are identical in all pools. A general three-compartment model has nine independent parameters, so two parameters remain undetermined.

In such cases essential information may still be obtained by a method introduced by Berman [47,277]. This method determines the ranges of parameter values which are compatible with the specific model proposed and the activity curves measured. These ranges are also limited by the fact that transfer constants cannot assume negative values. Using this method it is often found that, although the exact values of parameters cannot be determined, the range of physically possible parameter values is quite narrow, or even is absent in which case the proposed model is rejected. For example, if the protein is eliminated very slowly compared to the time needed for equilibration of $P(t)$ with $E_1(t)$ and $E_2(t)$ (cf. Fig. 4.3), the elimination rate as determined from exponential analysis will hardly be influenced by possible direct exchange of protein between $E_1(t)$ and $E_2(t)$.

Some information can be obtained from n-compartment linear models, irrespective of the number or arrangement of the extravascular pools. Such information is not directly applicable to quantification of protein release into plasma because, as shown in Table 4.1, calculation of $A(t)$ requires knowledge of the number of exponentials necessary to describe the disappearance curve after bolus injection. This number also defines a minimal number of compartments. Still these general methods offer useful checks by furnishing overall parameter values such as the sum of intra- and extravascular elimination rates and the total extravascular protein pool. Moreover, these methods require minimal a-priori physiological knowledge of the circulatory system studied. Because of its elegance and simplicity, the method of Nosslin [331] has been used increasingly frequent in the literature. Fig. 4.7 shows the plasma protein pool $P_b(t)$ and the total body pool $T_b(t) = P_b(t) + E_b(t)$ measured after intravascular bolus injection of one unit of protein at time t=0. The extravascular protein pool $E_b(t)$ may be subdivided in any number of extravascular sub-pools.

In practical applications of this method one mostly considers radiolabeled protein preparations and $T_b(t)$ is measured by subtracting urinary excretion of radioactivity from the total injected quantity of radioactivity or, in some cases, by whole-body counting techniques. Nosslin has shown that in this case we have (cf. Appendix):

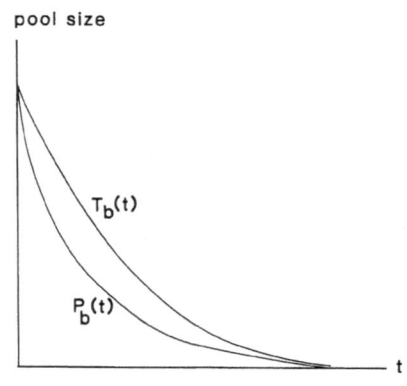

pool size

Fig 4.7 Integral method as used by Noss-lin, ref.331.

$$k_{tot} = 1/[\int_0^\infty P_b(\tau)d\tau]$$

$$(E/P)_s = [\int_0^\infty T_b(\tau)d\tau]/[\int_0^\infty P_b(\tau)d\tau] - 1 \qquad (4.18)$$

where k_{tot} is the total elimination constant, expressed as a fractional rate constant of $P(t)$, and $(E/P)_s$ is the steady-state ratio of extravascular to intravascular protein pools as discussed before.

As an example we consider the two-compartment model presented in Fig. 4.2. In that case we obtained: $P_b(t) = P_1 \exp(-k_1 t) + P_2 \exp(-k_2 t)$ or $k_{tot} = 1/(P_1/k_1 + P_2/k_2)$. From equation (4.8) we then find: $k_{tot} = FCR + k_e \cdot TER/(ERR+k_e) = FCR + k_e \cdot (E/P)_s$ which is indeed the total fractional catabolic rate constant related to the plasma pool.

Note that the result (4.18) has very general validity. The only conditions required are the linearity of the system and an intravascular input of protein.

If it can be assumed that only intravascular elimination of protein occurs, the curve $T_b(t)$ in Fig. 4.7 need no longer to be determined and all information can be obtained from the plasma curve $P_b(t)$. In that case we have (cf. Appendix):

$$\text{FCR} \quad = 1/[\int_0^\infty P_b(\tau)d\tau]$$

$$(E/P)_s = [\int_0^\infty \tau\, P_b(\tau)d\tau]/[\int_0^\infty P_b(\tau)d\tau]^2 - 1 \qquad (4.19)$$

$$\text{TER} \quad = -\,[\frac{d}{dt}P_b(t)]_{t=0} + \text{FCR}$$

where TER is the sum of fractional transcapillary escape rates
from the plasma to any number of extravascular compartments.

Use of equations (4.18) en (4.19) is complicated by the fact
that the contribution to the integral terms for $t \to \infty$, i.e. the
"tail" of the integrals, must somehow be estimated. Usually this
is done by exponential fitting of the last part of the plasma
curve, which makes the method to some extent equivalent to the
usual analysis in exponential terms.

4.3 Equivalence of different methods and formalisms

The purpose of this section is to give a short summary of the
methods used by different authors in quantitative studies of
circulating proteins and to stress the analogies between different formalisms and the representation adopted in the preceding
section.

A pharmacokinetic study, published by T. Teorell in 1937
[474], is cited [77] as the first application of compartmental
analysis to the circulatory system. Compartmental studies of
circulating proteins were started around 1950, after the introduction of techniques for labeling of proteins with radioactive
isotopes (cf. Section 5.3). It was soon realized that some early
methods used for analysis of plasma protein kinetics were based
upon invalid assumptions and could introduce considerable error.
Still these methods were widely used and even may be encountered
in the literature today. The best known of these pioneer methods
is explained in Fig. 4.8. This method is applied to biphasic
plama disappearance curves after intravascular bolus injection of
protein (cf. equation (4.5)):

$$P(t) = P_1 e^{-k_1 t} + P_2 e^{-k_2 t} + P_s \quad \text{with} \quad P_1, P_2, k_1, k_2 > 0.$$

A plot of $\ln[P(t)-P_s]$ versus time will approach to a straight line with a slope equal to the exponential constant with the lowest value, say k_2, and an intercept at the ordinate of $\ln P_2$. Knowing P_2, P_1 can be found from extrapolation of the rapid disappearance phase to $t=0$. It is assumed that the slow disappearance phase represents the phase of catabolic elimination of protein from the plasma, i.e. $FCR=k_2$, and the rapid disappearance phase represents the loss of protein from the plasma to an extravascular pool. The steady-state pool ratio $(P+E)_s/P_s$ is estimated as $(P_1+P_2)/P_2$. However, the slow disappearance phase reflects the combined effects of catabolic elimination from the plasma and reflux of protein from the extravascular space to the plasma. So, the fractional catabolic rate constant is underestimated, $FCR > k_2$, and the extravascular protein pool is overestimated.

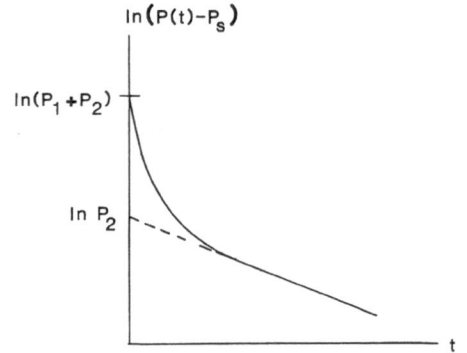

Fig 4.8 *Extrapolation method as used by Sterling, ref. 451.*

The first systematic analysis of experimentally obtained plasma protein curves in terms of a multi-compartment mamillary system was given in 1956 [301]. This study was based upon an earlier mathematical analysis [374]. Fig. 4.9 illustrates the formalism used in this study. The model is obviously equivalent to the system presented in Fig. 4.4 apart from the fact that elimination of protein is treated as unidirectional transport to an "excretion" pool, $X_2(t)$, which can be determined as a function of time by measurement of cumulative excretion of radioactivity

in urine and faeces. In case of intravascular catabolism and rapid excretion of radiolabel, FCR can be directly estimated from
the relation [85 , 83]:

$$FCR = u(t)/P(t) \qquad\qquad (4.20)$$

where u(t) is the excreted activity per hour (or per day) at time
t. In Fig. 4.9 we have $u(t) = \frac{d}{dt} X_2(t)$.

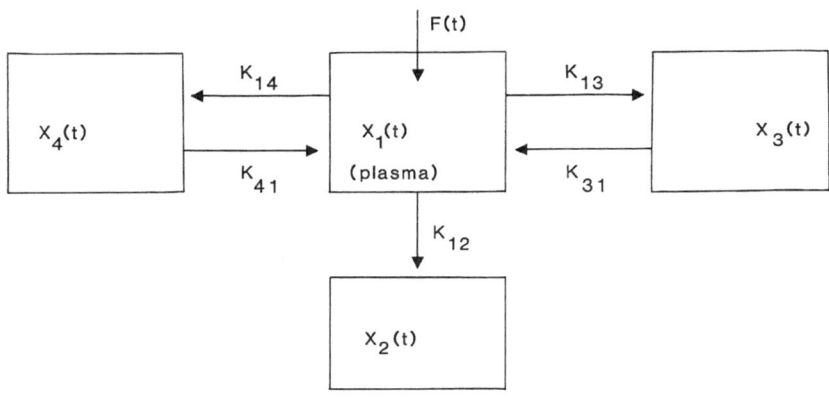

*Fig 4.9 The three-compartment system in its original
notation, ref.301.*

It was soon noted [277,361], however, that use of equation (4.20)
for calculation of FCR may introduce error because of accumulation of radioactive protein degradation products in the body.
This situation is shown in Fig. 4.10 (cf. also Fig. 4.6).

The excretion rate constant for radioactive degradation products of iodonated albumin in man is relatively constant [277]:
k_I=0.065 h^{-1}. As this value exceeds the FCR of albumin by more
than a factor of 10, only a small error will occur if I(t) is
neglected. For more rapidly catabolized proteins, however, substantial error may be introduced [139]. In such cases the iodine
pool I(t) may be estimated from cumulative urinary excretion
U(t):

$$U(t) = k_I \int_o^t I(\tau)d\tau \; ; \; I(t) = \frac{1}{k_T} \frac{d}{dt} U(t) \; (k_I = 0.065 \text{ h}^{-1}) \quad (4.21)$$

Some authors [85, 532, 202, 527] have considered models with diffusional exchange of protein between intra- and extravascular compartments. In such models, the rate of exchange of protein is determined by the difference between intra- and extravascular protein concentrations, $C_p(t)$ and $C_e(t)$, and a single permeability constant P which is equal for the transport in both directions. Fig. 4.11 presents the formalism for these models. Such a model is equivalent with the model presented in Fig. 4.2 without extra-vascular elimination of protein ($k_e=0$):

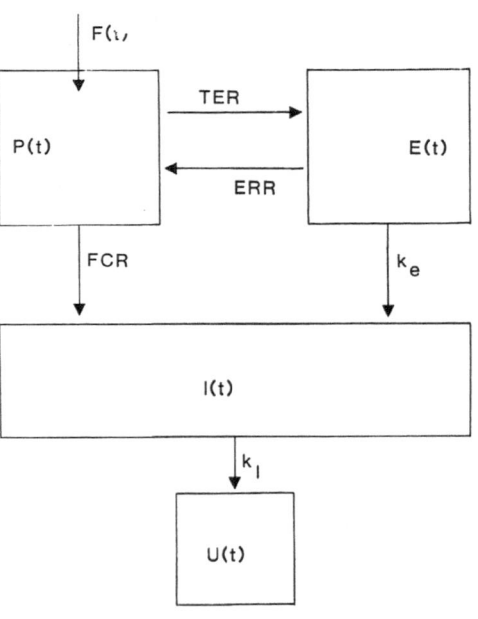

Fig 4.10 Two-compartment model with an added pool I(t) for iodinated protein degradation products.

$$\begin{aligned} P(t) &= V_p \, C_p(t) \\ E(t) &= V_e \, C_e(t) \qquad (4.22) \\ TER &= P/V_p \\ ERR &= P/V_e. \end{aligned}$$

The use of protein concentrations also inspired the so called "equilibrium-time" method for the determination of the ratio of pool sizes (cf. Fig. 4.12). For this method E(t) must be determined either by subtracting P(t)

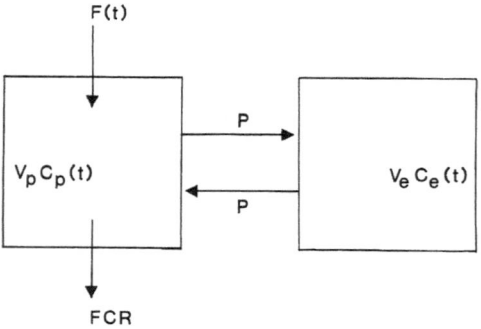

Fig 4.11 Two-compartment model with diffusional exchange of protein.

from whole-body counts [85] or by subtracting P(t), U(t) and I(t) (cf. Fig. 4.10) from the total dose of injected activity. The equilibrium time t_{eq} is defined as the time at which E(t) reaches its maximal value and there is no net transport of protein between P(t) and E(t). This implies that t_{eq} may also be defined as the time at which the slope of the plasma disappearance curve equals FCR. For the model of Fig. 4.11 this implies that $C_p(t_{eq}) = C_e(t_{eq})$ (cf. Fig. 4.12) and we have:

$$E(t_{eq})/P(t_{eq}) = [V_e C_e(t_{eq})]/[V_p C_p(t_{eq})] = V_e/V_p = E_s/P_s. \qquad (4.23)$$

This method offers the advantage of a much shorter period of observation than required for determination of exponential disappearance curves.

A number of authors have stressed the interpretation of transfer rate constants as reciprocal transit times. A linear transport process with a fractional transfer rate constant of $k(h^{-1})$ may be characterized by the fact that every molecule in the protein pool has a probability of magnitude k to be removed in the

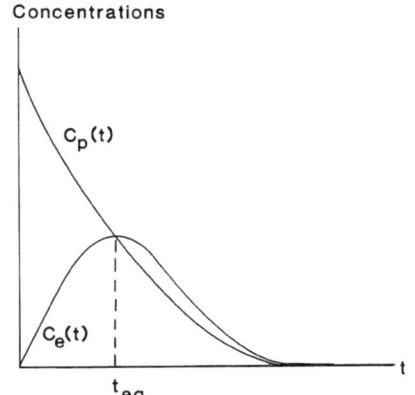

Fig 4.12 *Equilibrium-time method for the determination of the steady-state pool ratio, as used by Campbell, ref. 85.*

next hour. The mean time of sojourn of protein molecules in the pool will then be 1/k hours. The mean total life span of a molecule in the plasma pool will thus be 1/FCR hours, while the mean plasma transit time and the mean interstitial transit time will be respectively 1/TER and 1/ERR hours. One may also use the concept of the mean number of transit tours per molecule. For instance for albumin the mean plasma transit time is approximately 20 hours (TER = 0.05 h^{-1}) while the mean total life span in plasma (plasma sojourn time) is approximately 250 hours (FCR = 0.004 h^{-1}). These values imply that the mean number of transit tours per molecule of albumin will be approximately 13.

The concept of interstitial transit times was used in the "multi-pipe" model presented in Fig. 4.13. Instead of a few well-mixed extravascular compartments, one considers a large number of extravascular channels of which two are shown in Fig. 4.13. Each channel is characterized by a specific transit time. In the preceding section it was shown that a single extravascular pool, characterized by a single interstitial transit time 1/ERR,

results in the following expression: $E(t) = TER._0\int^t P(\tau)\exp(-ERR(t-\tau))d\tau$. In the multi-pipe model, this expression is replaced by: $E(t) = TER._0\int^t P(\tau) f(t-\tau)d\tau$, where the function $f(t)$ gives the fraction of transit times longer than t. The overall extravascular return rate of protein in this model (cf. Fig. 4.13) is given by:

$$\psi(t) = -(\frac{d}{dt}E(t) - TER.P(t))$$

$$= -TER\int_0^t P(\tau)\frac{d}{dt}f(t-\tau)d\tau$$

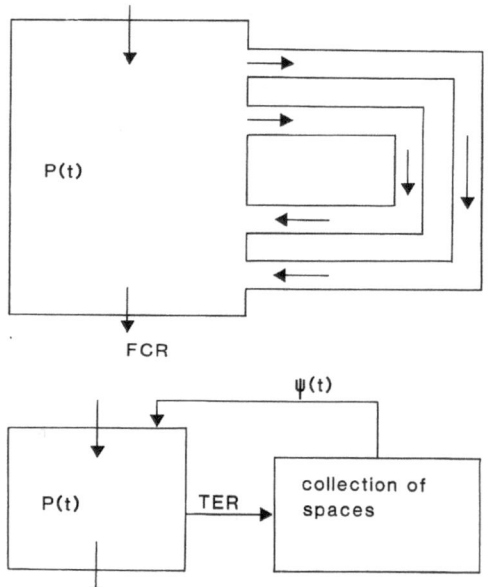

Fig 4.13 Multi-pipe model as used by Reeve, ref. 362.

Although this model offers a more attractive physiological picture of extravascular protein dynamics than a simple two- or three-compartment model, this advantage is lost as soon as it is used in exponential analysis of protein curves [464]. A tri-exponential disappearance curve $P_b(t)$, for instance, is compatible with a three-compartment model as presented in Fig. 4.3 with

$$E(t)=TER_1\int_0^t P(\tau)\exp[-ERR_1(t-\tau)]d\tau + TER_2\int_0^t P(\tau)\exp[-ERR_2(t-\tau)]d\tau$$

This implies that the general function f(t) has been reduced to a double-exponential function, i.e. a situation with two distinct extravascular pools with transit times $1/ERR_1$ and $1/ERR_2$. Thus, the multi-pipe model becomes equivalent to an n-compartment mammillary system as soon as the plasma disappearance curve $P_b(t)$ is approximated by an n-exponential function. The multi-pipe model illustrates that the introduction of physiologically realistic models, containing more parameters, is relatively fruitless as long as only a limited amount of information can be extracted from the experimental data. This is also true for so-called stochastic circulatory models in which it is assumed that the values of model parameters show stochastic fluctuations [77]. Although such fluctuations certainly occur, the accuracy of determination of plasma protein curves is insufficient for determination of the parameters characterizing these stochastic processes such as the standard deviation of fluctuations around the mean.

A simple graphical method for the determination of parameter values for two-compartment models is presented in Fig. 4.14.

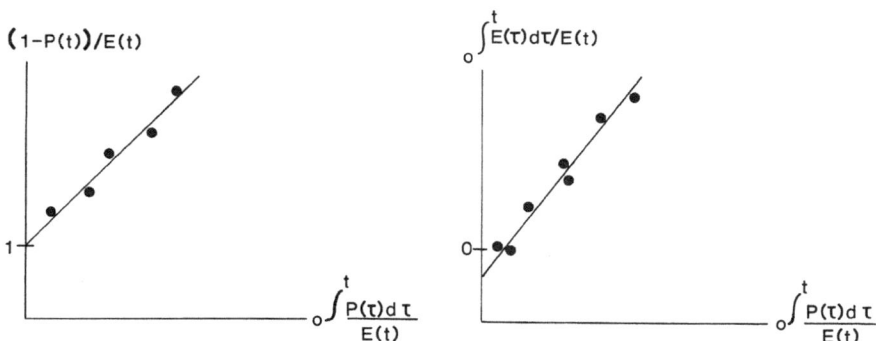

Fig 4.14   Integral method for short time intervals as used by Nosslin, ref.332.

From equation (4.11) we find for an intravascular bolus of one unit of protein:

$$1 = P(t) + (1-\frac{k_e}{ERR+k_e})E(t) + (FCR + \frac{k_e \cdot TER}{ERR+k_e}) \int_o^t P(\tau)\tau$$

or

$$\frac{1-P(t)}{E(t)} = (1 - \frac{k_e}{ERR+k_e}) + (FCR + \frac{k_e \cdot TER}{ERR+k_e}) \frac{\int_o^t P(\tau)d\tau}{E(t)} \tag{4.24}$$

Also, $E(t)$ must be equal to the net result of inflow and outflow: $E(t) = TER._o\int^t P(\tau)d\tau - (ERR+k_e)_o\int^t E(\tau)d\tau$,

or

$$\frac{\int_o^t E(\tau)d\tau}{E(t)} = -\frac{1}{ERR+k_e} + \frac{TER}{ERR+k_e} \frac{\int_o^t P(\tau)d\tau}{E(t)} \tag{4.25}$$

Fig. 4.14 shows how these relations are used in order to obtain the relevant parameters from the slopes and intercepts of two straight lines. The occurrence of extravascular elimination of protein ($k_e \neq 0$) is apparent from the fact that the line in the left hand plot passes below the point $(0,1)$. The method is claimed to be applicable over short time intervals. It can also be easily extended to the model presented in Fig. 4.10 [332].

An elegant double-label technique for the determination of FCR can also be applied for short time intervals. This method is based on simultaneous injection of ^{125}I-iodide and ^{131}I-albumin.

For a linear system we have (cf. equation 4.2):

$$^{131}I(t) = \int_o^t F(\tau) \, ^{125}I_b(t-\tau)d\tau$$

where $^{131}I(t)$ is the plasma pool of ^{131}I-iodide released from ^{131}I-albumin, $F(t)$ is the rate of release of ^{131}I-iodide into plasma and $I_b(t)$ is the response curve to the bolus injection of ^{125}I-iodide. If the breakdown of albumin occurs intravascularly, i.e. $F(t) = FCR \cdot {}^{131}P(t)$, where $^{131}P(t)$ is the plasma pool of ^{131}I-albumin, one obtains:

$$^{131}I(t) = FCR \int_o^t {}^{131}P(\tau) \, {}^{125}I_b(t-\tau)d\tau$$

This equation allows determination of FCR because $^{131}I(t)$ and

^{131}P(t) can be measured in plasma after separation of ^{131}I-iodide and ^{131}I-albumin by gel filtration and ^{125}I$_b$(t) can be measured simultaneously. The only conditions used in this method are the linearity of the system and absence of extravascular breakdown of protein. Assumptions about the number or arrangement of extravascular pools are not used [55].

The same is true for a method which is based on the characterization of the extravascular response as a convolution integral of the plasma curve [508]:

$$E(t) = \int_0^t P(\tau) \, G(t-\tau) d\tau. \qquad (4.26)$$

Comparison of this integral with equation (4.2) shows that the transfer function G(t) is essentially the response function to an extravascular bolus injection of one unit of protein. This response function is completely determined in less than one week which is a considerable shorter period of time than needed for complete characterization of disappearance curves of slowly catabolized proteins such as albumin, fibrinogen or immunoglobulins. The function G(t) can be calculated from direct measurements of P(t) and E(t) during a few days. Knowing G(t), the other relevant parameters are calculated from the relations:

$$TER = G(t=0);$$

$$(E/P)_s = \int_0^\infty G(\tau) d\tau.$$

Fig.4.15 presents a method for estimation of model parameter values by comparison of plasma protein kinetics after bolus injection and during continuous infusion of protein. For the initial exponential disappearance constant

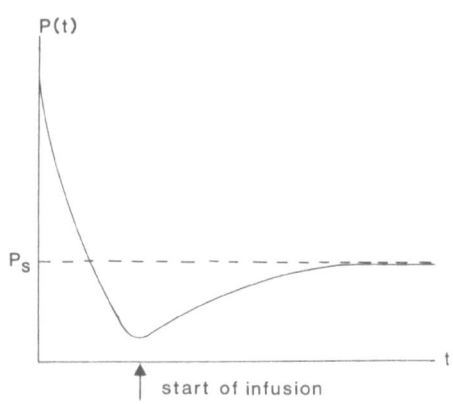

Fig 4.15 Combination of intra-vascular bolus injection and constant-rate infusion of protein.

$k_{t=0}$ one has:

$$k_{t=0} = FCR + TER$$

The subsequent infusion is maintained at a constant rate of F units of protein per hour until a steady state is reached. In the steady state we have:

$$F = FCR \cdot P_s \quad \text{or} \quad FCR = F/P_s.$$

Using these relations, FCR and TER may be estimated without further assumptions about the number or configuration of extravascular compartments. If TER is much smaller than FCR, the steady state reached in Fig. 4.15 may be only apparent. In that case one has essentially a one-compartment model and the extravascular compartment, instead of being saturated, may hardly contain protein. In that case the apparent steady state is characterized by $F = (FCR + TER) \cdot P_s$.

Sudden depletion of the plasma protein pool has also been used as a means of estimating circulatory parameter values. This method is shown in Fig. 4.16.

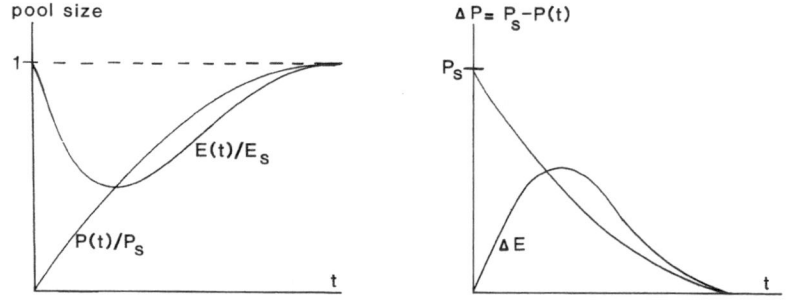

Fig 4.16 Effect of sudden depletion of the plasma protein pool at time t = 0.

The system is assumed to be in a steady state with a plasma protein pool P_s and an extravascular protein pool E_s. At time t=0, the plasma protein pool is suddenly depleted and subsequent return to normal values is observed. Examples of such depletion are the elimination of plasma haptoglobin after intravenous infusion of hemoglobin [333]; depletion of circulating immuno-globulins by intravenous infusion of antigen [170] or removal of plasminogen by intravenous infusion of streptokinase [323]. It is easily verified (cf. Appendix) that the differences $\Delta P = P_s - P(t)$ and $\Delta E = E_s - E(t)$ in Fig. 4.16 can be described by equations similar to the response curves after a bolus injection of protein:

$$\Delta P = P_s - P(t) = P_1 e^{-k_1 t} + P_2 e^{-k_2 t}$$
$$\Delta E = E_s - E(t) = R_1 e^{-k_1 t} + R_2 e^{-k_2 t} \qquad (4.28)$$

where P_1, P_2, R_1, R_2, k_1 and k_2 are given by equation (4.6).

A similar method could be based on sudden changes in the rate of protein release into plasma. Examples of such situations are the disappearance and reappearance of plasma coagulation factors during oral anticoagulant therapy and disappearance of tissue-specific proteins from plasma after surgical removal of tumours or diseased organs. If it is assumed that the input function $F(t)$ of protein into plasma shows a sudden change:

$$F(t) = F_s = \text{constant for } t < 0$$
$$F(t) = F_1 = \text{constant for } t \geq 0$$

one finds for a two-compartment model (cf. Appendix)

$$\Delta P = P_s - P(t) = Q_1 + Q_2 - Q_1 e^{-k_1 t} - Q_2 e^{-k_2 t} \qquad (4.29)$$

with $Q_1 = (F_s - F_1)P_1/k_1$; $Q_2 = (F_s - F_1)P_2/k_2$; P_1, P_2, k_1, k_2 given by equation (4.6).

Table 4.2 presents a comparison of results obtained by appli-cation of different methods on identical data. Considering the equivalence of different methods, it is not surprising that identical results are mostly obtained.

Table 4.2 : Comparison of different methods for analysis of
protein kinetics in man.

Ref.	Protein	Method	number of exp.	$FCR(h^{-1})\pm CV(\%)$	$(E/P)_s\pm CV(\%)$
[100]	albumin	A	11	0.0043 ± 13	1.4 ± 21
[100]	albumin	B	6	0.0037 ± 13	
[100]	albumin	C	6		1.2 ± 23
[37]	albumin	A	20	0.0050 ± 14	1.3 ± 15
[37]	albumin	B	20	0.0049 ± 17	
[37]	albumin	C	20		1.2 ± 12
[99]	IgG	A	11	0.0028 ± 25	0.85 ± 27
[99]	IgG	B	9	0.0025 ± 28	
[99]	IgG	C	9		1.0 ± 15
[15]	IgG	C	6		0.92 ± 14
[15]	IgG	D	6		0.89 ± 9
[8]	IgG	A	14	0.0032 ± 36	
[8]	IgG	E	12	0.0028 ± 52	
[465]	fibrinogen	A	12	0.010 ± 7	0.19 ± 23
[465]	fibrinogen	B	12	0.010 ± 11	
[241]	α_1-antitrypsin	A	7	0.014 ± 11	1.1 ± 17
[241]	α_1-antitrypsin	B	7	0.013 ± 13	
[241]	α_1-antitrypsin	C	7		1.1 ± 11
[241]	α_1-antitrypsin	E	7	0.013 ± 11	1.2 ± 13
[84]	low density lipoprotein(LDL)	A	7	0.012 ± 36	0.41 ± 23
[84]	LDL	B	8	0.012 ± 36	
[84]	LDL	C	9		0.54 ± 17
[84]	LDL	E	9		0.43 ± 23

A: multi-exponential analysis (Matthews '57)

B: measurement of urinary excretion (Berson '57)

C: equilibrium-time method (Campbell '56)

D: integral-method for long time intervals (Nosslin '64)

E: integral-method for short time intervals (Nosslin '73).

Method E has recently been used more frequently because it can be applied for short time intervals and offers a simple graphical check on the ocurrence of extravascular elimination.

Results as shown in Table 4.2 may be compared with results obtained by independent techniques. The rate of protein synthesis has been measured with so called "pulse-labeling" techniques [417]. A radiolabeled precursor substance is injected into the plasma and incorporated in protein molecules by normal biosynthesis. The best-known methods are based upon ^{14}C-arginine, either directly injected or in vivo synthesized from injected ^{14}C-carbonate [290,363]. The labeled arginine is used for simultaneous production of protein and urea in liver cells. The rate of protein synthesis is estimated by assuming that the labeled fraction of the quantity of urea produced must be equal to the labeled fraction of protein produced in the same time interval. Total steady-state production of urea can be estimated from urinary excretion. Production of labeled urea is obtained by adding excreted radioactivity to the amount of circulating ^{14}C-urea. The latter is calculated from plasma ^{14}C-urea concentration and urea distribution space. The quantity of labeled protein produced is determined in plasma and corrected for the loss due to extravasation and elimination by measuring the disappearance curve of ^{131}I-labeled protein over the same time interval. Experiments as presented in Table 4.2 were performed in steady-state conditions, which implies that FCR must equal the fractional synthesis rate constant i.e. the quantity of protein produced per hour (or per day) expressed as a fraction of the steady-state plasma pool. Further refinements in measurement of protein synthesis have mainly been developed in studies on intracellular protein turnover [539]. A number of problems in pulse labeling can be avoided by continuous infusion - instead of bolus injection - of precursors [450]. Uncertainties about the mixing times of precursor pools or about the interpretation of urea kinetics can be eliminated in this way. Other uncertainties however remain, such as possible breakdown of urea by the intestinal flora or the existence of separate precursor pools for urea and protein [472]. Another improvement consists of the introduction of nonradioactive isotopes which can be measured by optical emission spectroscopy or by mass spectroscopy. These techniques permit more studies in volunteers because radiation hazards are avoided. The precursors most frequently used in such studies are ^{15}N-glycine and ^{15}N-ammonium. The isotopic enrichment of the hepatic protein precursor pool may be estimated from the urinary production of ^{15}N-hippuric acid [450].

As a rule, values of FCR estimated from various methods for the determination of protein synthesis rates are in good agreement with values of FCR obtained from the methods presented in Table 4.2. This is also true for rates of synthesis as estimated by direct measurement of changes in circulating protein mass after administration of synthesis-blocking agents in the so-called mass balance method [365]. As discussed in Section 3.3 this is not true for values of $(E/P)_s$. Direct measurement of extravascular albumin pools has demonstrated discrepancies. In a number of studies, significantly larger values of $(E/P)_s$ than indicated in Table 4.2 were found.

4.4   Limitations and possibilities in quantification of continuing in-vivo release of protein

In this section we return to the problem of quantification of proteins released into the circulation. As shown in Section 4.2, the information needed for such quantification can be obtained by studying disappearance curves after a bolus injection of protein (cf. Table 4.1). "Injections" of protein may often occur in clinical situations. Examples are the transient elevations of plasma levels of tissue enzymes due to leakage of enzymes from damaged tissues (cf. Chapter 6), transient increases in the rate of synthesis of "acute phase" proteins after trauma (cf. Chapter 7) and therapeutic infusion of protein preparations in patients with coagulation factor deficiencies (cf. Chapter 8). It is of importance to verify whether such naturally occurring inputs of protein can be used, instead of bolus injections, in order to obtain the information needed for quantification of protein release.

Let us first consider a one-compartment model with a transient input of F(t) units of protein per hour, shown in Fig. 4.17. For first-order elimination with a fractional catabolic rate constant FCR we have:

$$\frac{d}{dt} P(t) = -FCR.P(t) - F(t)$$

(4.30)

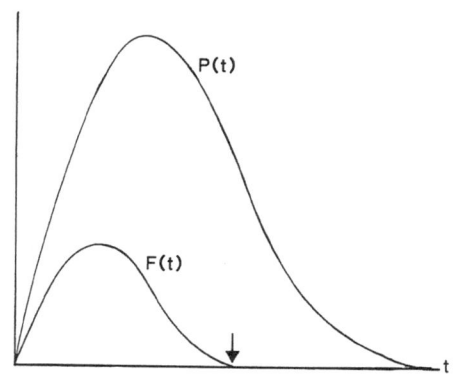

The individual value of FCR in the patient or experimental animal studied is usually not known. So the problem is to find both, F(t) and FCR, from the plasma curve P(t).

Fig 4.17   *Transient input of protein in a one-compartment model.*

If one has a true release function F(t) and a true elimination constant FCR, one may take an arbitrary constant FCR' and consider the release function F'(t) defined by:

$$F'(t) = F(t) + (FCR - FCR')P(t)$$

(4.31)

Substitution of this expression into equation (4.30) yields:

$$\frac{d}{dt} P(t) = -FCR'.P(t) + F'(t)$$

which implies that the observed change in time of P(t) may equally well be explained by a different input function and a different elimination constant. It is impossible to identify both the correct value of FCR and the correct input function F(t) from analysis of the plama curve P(t) of a single protein.

We have now considered a one-compartment situation and it will be clear that the lack of information becomes even worse in a two-compartment system. In fact it can be shown that instead of the one-parameter (FCR') family of input functions (4.31) we have in that case a three-parameter family of functions. This implies that parameters such as the transcapillary escape rate constant and the extravascular return rate constant are undetermined, just like the elimination constant FCR.

This inherent limitation in the information that can be obtained from measurement of P(t) can be overcome if it can be assumed that beyond a certain time - indicated in Fig. 4.17 - no further input of protein occurs. The solution of equation (4.26) can be written (cf. equation (4.2)):

$$P(t) = e^{-FCR \cdot t} \int_{0}^{t} e^{FCR \cdot \tau} F(\tau) d\tau$$

which implies that if F(t) = 0 for $t > t_e$ we have:

$$P(t) = K \cdot e^{-FCR \cdot t} \qquad K = constant, \ t > t_e$$

Thus, the correct value of FCR can be obtained from an exponential fit on the "tail" of the plasma curve P(t). In fact this procedure has been often applied in the literature but the period of protein release has mostly been underestimated in these studies. Physiological release functions usually show considerable tailing and even a small amount of residual release of protein may cause considerable error in estimated values of FCR [527].

The difficulty just mentioned may be overcome if a trace amount of labeled protein is injected during the period of observation. In this case FCR may be estimated independently by one of the methods discussed in the preceding section, for instance by use of the relation $FCR = u(t)/P^*(t)$, where u(t) is the radioactivity excreted per hour and $P^*(t)$ is the plasma radioactivity. This method was used in order to measure the effect of hormones on albumin synthesis rates [178],and the effect of myocardial infarction on the catabolic rate of creatine kinase [440].

Another possibility to overcome these limitations is offered when two proteins are released simultaneously and in a fixed proportion ρ into the plasma:

$$A_2(t) = \rho \cdot A_1(t)$$

$$A_1(t) = P_1(t) + FCR_1 \int_{0}^{t} P_1(\tau) d\tau \qquad (4.32)$$

$$A_2(t) = P_2(t) + FCR_2 \int_0^t P_2(\tau)d\tau$$

Eliminating $A_1(t)$ and $A_2(t)$ from these relations one obtains:

$$P_2(t) + FCR_2 \int_0^t P_2(\tau)d\tau = \rho.P_1(t) + \rho.FCR_1 \int_0^t P_1(\tau)d\tau \quad (4.33)$$

By measurement of $P_1(t)$ and $P_2(t)$ for $t=t_1,t_2...t_n$, the parameters ρ, FCR_1, and FCR_2 can be obtained. To this end the parameter values are adjusted in order to minimize the difference between the lefthand side and the righthand side of equation (4.33).

This method, based on simultaneous release of two different proteins, can also be applied to two-compartment models. Instead of equation (4.33) one then obtains:

$$P_2(t) + TER \int_0^t e^{-ERR(t-\tau)} P_2(\tau)d\tau + FCR_2 \int_0^t P_2(\tau)d\tau =$$

$$\rho.P_1(t) + \rho.TER \int_0^t e^{-ERR(t-\tau)}P_1(\tau)d\tau + \rho.FCR_1 \int_0^t P_1(\tau)d\tau \quad (4.34)$$

where it has been assumed that values of TER and ERR are identical for both proteins. Equation (4.34) has been used, in a different form, to obtain the parameter values of ρ, FCR_1, FCR_2, TER and ERR for the myocardial enzymes CK and HBDH released in patients with acute myocardial infarction [527]. However, the fitting procedure in this case is complicated by the non-linear terms and the error in obtained parameter values is large because of the large number of parameters to be estimated.

A special situation arises if one of the elimination constants, say FCR_2, has a low value and the time interval of fitting is short enough to keep the eliminated fraction of the slowly catabolized enzyme relatively small. If these conditions are fulfilled a fixed mean value for FCR_2 may be used, neglecting variation between individuals. Thus the problem is reduced to a two-parameter (ρ and FCR_1) fitting problem. Further details of this method will be given in Chapter 6.

CHAPTER 5

SOURCES OF ERROR IN QUANTIFICATION OF CIRCULATING PROTEINS

5.1 Introduction

Systematic investigation of the turnover and distribution of circulating proteins was made possible by the introduction of radiolabeled protein preparations. Indeed, the ideal molecular probe seemed to be discovered: indistinguishable from native molecules in the physico-chemical properties determining biological elimination and distribution, but easily and accurately detectable. The high accuracy of measurement stimulated multicompartment analysis of disappearance curves. High values for transcapillary escape rates of proteins, as reported in some early studies with radiolabeled proteins, did not cause any doubts about experimental validity.

In 1953, however, it was noticed that the measured half-lifes for the disappearance of radiolabeled albumin and IgG varied respectively from 10-20 days to 7-27 days [50]. Moreover, the reported half-lifes of ^{131}I-albumin appeared to be dependent on the period of observation and on the degree of labeling of the protein. It was concluded that labeled protein molecules may show abnormal behaviour.

As will be presently discussed, the difficulties can be attributed to several causes. Firstly, it is known that even if an ideal label is used, i.e. if the labeled molecules cannot be distinguished from native ones, the behaviour of tracers does not necessarily reflect the behaviour of the unlabeled bulk of protein. This is true for the rate of elimination as well as for the transcapillary escape rate. Secondly, the process of purification and/or labeling of protein may induce molecular changes that have distinct effects on the elimination rates, the altered molecules usually being eliminated more rapidly. Such rapid elimination of fractions of damaged molecules has often been erroneously inter-

preted as extravasation of protein. Thirdly, recycling of bio-
sythetic labels such as ^{15}N-, ^{14}C- or ^{35}S-aminoacids, or accumulation of labeled degradation products in the body, may invalidate the comparison between in vivo behaviour of label and
protein.

In addition to the mentioned artefacts, which may cause gross
errors, we come across inaccuracies in parameter values used in
the calculations and experimental errors in protein determinations. The effect of these errors is largely dependent on the
period of observation and the elimination rate of the specific
protein to be quantified.

Sources of error have often resulted in incorrect conclusions
about the circulatory system. In the final section of this chapter this will be illustrated with examples from literature concerning the study of the appropriate circulatory model for the
distribution and turnover of proteins in the dog.

5.2 Hazards in estimating circulatory parameters from tracer kinetics

In this section an ideal tracer will be considered, in other
words it is assumed that the presence of label does not affect
the molecular properties that are relevant to the in vivo distribution and elimination of protein.

As discussed in the preceding chapter, a common procedure for
determining circulatory parameters consists of analysis of disappearance curves of plasma radioactivity after intravenous
injection of labeled protein. If the labeled molecules are indeed
indistinguishable from native molecules, the elimination rates of
both molecular species must be proportional to their presence in
the plasma:

$$\frac{dP^*}{dt} \Big/ \frac{dP}{dt} = P^*/P$$

where P^* is the plasma pool of labeled protein and P is the plasma pool of the unlabeled bulk of protein.

The value of P is not influenced by the minute quantity of added labeled protein, and we have

$$\frac{1}{P} \frac{dP}{dt} = - FCR \quad \text{or} \quad \frac{dP^*}{dt} = - FCR.P^*$$

This means that the tracer will be eliminated by a first-order process with a fractional elimination rate constant equal to FCR. If the value of P remains relatively constant during the period of observation, the value of FCR will remain also constant even if the protein considered has in fact a concentration-dependent FCR, such as for instance albumin (cf. Section 3.4). Thus, a departure of first-order elimination for the bulk of protein will not be apparent from tracer kinetics. One actually measures the fractional catabolic rate constant for the given bulk concentration of protein.

Transcapillary escape rates obtained in tracer experiments may also be different from the corresponding rates for bulk proteins. Compartmental analysis of such data is based upon relations of the type:

$$J^* = TER . P^*$$

in which J^* is the transcapillary tracer flux and TER is the transcapillary escape rate constant.

However, it follows from general thermodynamical principles that J^* will also be influenced by the presence of the bulk of protein. In fact we have the following relation [126]:

$$J^* = TER . P^* + L . P$$

in which the so-called cross-coefficient L only disappears when the labeled as well as the native molecules are diluted to such extent that interaction between both species is negligible. For the normal bulk concentrations of protein, however, a flow of unlabeled molecules will also drag along some labeled molecules, and consequently L cannot be neglected. As a rule, L is much smaller than TER [152], but the term L.P may still have a considerable effect on J^* because P is several orders of magnitude larger than P^*. This problem can only be solved rigorously by using two different ideal tracers [251].

For low molecular weight tracers, several authors have studied the influence of cross-effects in transfer through membranes [152,112,483]. For labeled proteins, however, systematic studies have not been made. This should be kept in mind when appraising puzzling observations such as concentration-dependent transcapillary escape rate constants or discrepancies in transfer rates found after injection of proteins into plasma or after depletion of the plasma protein pool [170].

The problem of cross-diffusional drag not only concerns tracer fluxes, but it may also affect transfer rates of other circulating proteins. According to the thermodynamical principle just mentioned, the diffusional flux of a certain substance may be affected by transfer of all other substances in the system. This implies, for instance, that the normal steady-state transcapillary flow of albumin might influence the rate of extravasation of circulating tissue enzymes.

5.3 Errors caused by purification and labeling of proteins

Proteins can be labeled by in-vitro techniques applied to purified protein preparations or by incorporation of labeled aminoacids through biosynthesis. The second method has the risk of re-utilization of label and has produced spuriously long plasma protein half-lifes [417]. The fact that in vitro labeled ^{131}I-albumin was eliminated more rapidly from the plasma than biosynthetically labeled albumin, was originally considered as proof for artefacts in the latter method [451]. Subsequently it was demonstrated, however, that most preparations of ^{131}I-albumin contained variable fractions of rapidly degrading components, probably as a result of self-irradiation damage [50,288,159]. In this respect it must be pointed out that even if the preparation as a whole does not contain more than a single atom of iodine per molecule of protein, the statistical distribution of label implies that some molecules must contain larger number of iodine atoms. Moreover, if for example 5% of the molecules in such a preparation contains 3 iodine atoms per molecule, this fraction containes 15% of total radioactivity. So, the presence of rapidly degraded fractions of protein can readily be explained. Several authors have attempted to determine the changes in the protein molecule that cause rapid in vivo elimination. The inability to characterize these changes by electrophoretic, chromatographic and ultracentrifugal separation techniques has led to the conclusion that even very subtle molecular changes may have distinct effects on in vivo elimination rates [417]. These molecular changes are not necessarily induced by the label proper but they may be the result of the purification procedure. Examination of two different albumin preparations, one prepared by alcohol fractionation and the other by salt fractionation, showed that both contain more than 90% of monomeric albumin, as proved with paper-, immuno- and moving boundary electrophoresis, gel filtration and ultracentrifugation. But after simultaneously injecting $^{131}I-$ and ^{125}I-labeled mixtures of the two preparations in volunteers, the preparation obtained by alcohol fractionation was eliminated more rapidly, irrespective of the applied label [393]. The inadequancy of physico-chemical separation techniques to detect such labile protein fractions resulted in the introduction of biological screening techniques [289]: after intravenously injecting protein preparations in experimental animals, the remaining fraction of protein is harvested from the plasma and used for experimentation.

Rapidly eliminated fractions have also been observed after intravenous injection of enzymes, as alkaline phosphatase[95],AST [512], LDH-5 [358], and human clotting factor VIII [342]. Indications of this phenomenon are the different values for plasma volume calculated from dilution of injected enzymes. Intravenous injection of purified preparations of CK(MM), CK(MB) and CK(BB) in dogs resulted in plasma volumes of respectively 67 ± 5 ml/kg, 78 ± 7 ml/kg and 104 ± 10 ml/kg (mean $\pm$ SEM, n = 6) [359]. This

indicates that these preparations contained increasingly large
fractions of damaged molecules; although still enzymatically
active, these molecules must have been eliminated almost instan-
taneously. It is interesting that the temperature-dependent
instability of CK isoenzymes seems related to the in vivo elimination rate. In the order CK(MM), CK(MB), CK(BB) these enzymes
are eliminated more rapidly and also show decreased temperature
stability. Simultaneous injection of AST, MDH and ALT in rabbits
also demonstrated different plasma volumes of respectively 32 $\pm$ 3
ml/kg, 40 $\pm$ 4 ml/kg and 23 $\pm$ 3 ml/kg (mean $\pm$ SE, n = 7) [11].
In a recent study precautions were taken to minimize the possible
causes of damage to enzyme molecules. A non-purified enzyme
preparation was obtained from anoxic incubation of tissue without
mechanical disruption of cells. Indeed, almost identical values
were found for the plasma volumes in dogs calculated from dilution of CK, LDH, AST and ALT, respectively 51 $\pm$ 1.4 ml/kg, 50 $\pm$
1.3 ml/kg, 47 $\pm$ 1.1 ml/kg and 47.4 $\pm$ 0.8 ml/kg (mean $\pm$ SEM, n =
10) [507].

Molecular alterations as mentioned thusfar always resulted in
accelerated in vivo elimination of proteins. However, there are
also some reports on molecular changes leading to prolonged in
vivo survival. In dogs acetylation of LDH produces a lower rate
of elimination [30]. As mentioned in Section 2.7, it was recently
shown that the M-subunit of CK may be changed by a heat-labile
factor in plasma and this change also results in slower elimination. These examples of enhanced in vivo stability are scarce and
when different elimination rates are observed for different protein preparations, it is usually assumed that the behaviour of
native molecules is best approximated by the slowly eliminated
preparation.

There are many examples in which the rapid initial disappearance phase, caused by a fraction of damaged protein molecules,
was interpreted as a distributional effect causing conspiciously
high values for transcapillary escape rates. To ascertain whether
biphasic disappearance curves as reported in literature may indeed reflect the effect of extravasation of protein, use can be
made of Table 5.1. The data in this table have been obtained as

Table 5.1 Biphasic disappearance of proteins from plasma.

FCR (h^{-1})	TER = 0.01 h^{-1}			TER = 0.03 h^{-1}			TER = 0.05 h^{-1}			TER = 0.07 h^{-1}		
	P_1	k_1	k_2	P_2	k_1	k_2	P_1	k_1	k_2	P_1	k_1	k_2
0.002	0.55	0.021	0.001	0.52	0.061	0.001	0.51	0.101	0.001	0.51	0.141	0.001
0.004	0.60	0.022	0.002	0.53	0.062	0.002	0.52	0.102	0.002	0.51	0.142	0.002
0.006	0.64	0.023	0.002	0.55	0.063	0.003	0.53	0.103	0.003	0.52	0.143	0.003
0.008	0.69	0.025	0.003	0.57	0.064	0.004	0.54	0.104	0.004	0.53	0.144	0.004
0.010	0.72	0.026	0.004	0.58	0.065	0.005	0.55	0.105	0.005	0.54	0.145	0.005
0.020	0.85	0.034	0.006	0.66	0.072	0.008	0.60	0.111	0.009	0.57	0.151	0.009
0.030	0.92	0.043	0.007	0.72	0.079	0.011	0.64	0.117	0.013	0.61	0.157	0.013
0.040	0.94	0.052	0.008	0.78	0.086	0.014	0.69	0.124	0.016	0.64	0.163	0.017
0.050	0.96	0.062	0.008	0.82	0.094	0.016	0.72	0.131	0.019	0.67	0.169	0.021
0.060	0.97	0.072	0.008	0.85	0.102	0.018	0.76	0.138	0.022	0.70	0.176	0.024
0.070	0.98	0.081	0.009	0.88	0.111	0.019	0.79	0.146	0.024	0.72	0.183	0.027
0.080	0.99	0.091	0.009	0.90	0.120	0.020	0.81	0.154	0.026	0.75	0.191	0.029
0.090	0.99	0.101	0.009	0.92	0.129	0.021	0.83	0.162	0.028	0.77	0.198	0.032
0.100	0.99	0.111	0.009	0.93	0.138	0.022	0.85	0.171	0.029	0.79	0.206	0.034
0.200	1.00	0.211	0.010	0.98	0.234	0.026	0.95	0.262	0.038	0.91	0.292	0.048
0.300	1.00	0.310	0.010	0.99	0.333	0.027	0.97	0.358	0.042	0.95	0.386	0.055
0.400	1.00	0.410	0.010	0.99	0.432	0.028	0.99	0.456	0.044	0.97	0.482	0.058
0.500	1.00	0.510	0.010	1.00	0.532	0.028	0.99	0.555	0.045	0.98	0.580	0.060

Disappearance of proteins - intravenously injected at time t=0 - is given by $P(t)=P_1\exp(-k_1t) +P_2\exp(-k_2t)$ with $P_2=1-P_1$. Values of k_1 and k_2 are expressed in $hour^{-1}$. Extravascular and intravascular protein pools are assumed to be of equal magnitude (see text).

follows. For proteins with molecular weights above M = 40,000 available information (cf. Chapter 9) shows that transcapillary escape rate constants (TER) in man are 0.01-0.07 h^{-1} under normal conditions. For such proteins, higher values of TER are only found under pathological conditions, e.g. hypertension [348]. For most proteins with molecular weights between M = 40,000 and M = 200,000, the extravascular protein pool roughly equals the plasma protein pool. Using these data the parameters P_1, P_2, k_1 and k_2 of the biphasic disappearance curve $P(t) = P_1 \exp(-k_1 t) + P_2 \exp(-k_2 t)$ were calculated from equation (4.6) for a range of FCR = 0.002 - 0.5 h^{-1}, TER = 0.01-0.07 h^{-1} and TER/ERR = $(E/P)_s$ = 1. From the coefficients P_1 and P_2 = 1 - P_1 it can be concluded that the disappearance curve will become essentially monophasic if FCR ≈ 0.1 h^{-1}. For values of TER = 0.01 h^{-1}, as reported for IgG and HBDH (cf. Chapter 9) this is even true if FCR > 0.02 h^{-1}. Thus a well-defined biphasic disappearance will only be observed for slowly eliminated enzymes. Table 5.1 can also be used to estimate FCR if only values of P_1, k_1 and k_2 are reported.

5.4 Accuracy in calculation of cumulative protein release

In this section it will be assumed that an initial steady state is disturbed by a process, starting at time t=0, resulting in a transient increase of the rate of protein entrance into plasma. Such increased release might be effected by intravenous infusion of proteins, increased synthesis of proteins in the liver, enhanced leakage of tissue proteins from damaged cells etc. In all these cases the problem is to estimate cumulative release of protein into plasma from serial measurements of plasma protein concentrations $C_p(t)$, t=t_1, t_2, t_3....,t_n.

As discussed in Chapter 4 this problem can be solved straightforwardly if the plasma response curve to an intravascular bolus injection of protein is known. However, it will be assumed that such information is not available. This implies that a specific circulatory model is needed and it is assumed that a two-compartment model, without extravascular elimination of enzyme, can be used. From equation (4.10) it follows that cumulative release of protein up to time t is given by:

$$A(t) = P(t) + E(t) + FCR \cdot \int_0^t P(\tau) d\tau$$

$$= V_p(t) \overline{C}_p(t) + TER \int_0^t V_p(\tau) \overline{C}_p(\tau) e^{-ERR(t-\tau)} d\tau + FCR \int_0^t V_p(\tau) \overline{C}_p(\tau) d\tau \tag{5.1}$$

where $V_p(t)$ and $C_p(t)$ respectively are the plasma volume and the plasma protein concentration at time t, while the second and the third term respectively give the extravasated and the eliminated quantities of protein. The bar added to $C_p(t)$ indicates that the plasma protein concentration must be corrected for the normal steady-state concentration C_s:

$$\overline{C}_p(t) = C_p(t) - C_s \tag{5.2}$$

This implies that A(t) does not include the normal steady-state release of protein but gives the extra release of protein due to the process started at t=0. If there is only transient extra release of protein and plasma protein concentrations can be measured up to a time t_s at which $C_p(t)$ has returned to its normal value C_s, total release may be calculated from the expression:

$$A_{tot} = FCR \cdot \int_0^{t_s} V_p(\tau) \overline{C}_p(\tau) d\tau \tag{5.3}$$

Equation (5.3) can be easily understood because the total quantity of protein entering the plasma will eventually be eliminated again from the plasma.

Values of A(t), as calculated from equation (5.1), are subject to error from various sources. Experimental scatter in determinations of plasma protein concentrations $C_p(t)$ will obviously cause error in A(t). However, this error may be kept within reasonable limits by use of multiple determinations. In most practical applications, use of duplicate determinations is sufficient to reduce this error to 2-4%.

A larger error may be introduced by the correction of $C_p(t)$ for the normal steady state plasma concentration C_s. Plasma protein concentrations are often already increased before the first plasma sample is obtained and may remain elevated for a long period of time. In such casus, no individual estimate of C_s can be obtained and a fixed mean value must be used. This implies that C_s may contain error due to variation between individuals. Healthy control persons usually show normally distributed values of C_s for most plasma proteins with variations of 10-20% (SD) [417,529]. Circulating tissue enzymes show skew (lognormal) distributions of C_s. For some enzymes this is more pronounced than for others. For instance for AST and ALT, the mean value of C_s is exceeded by 100% or more in one out of five persons, while for HBDH such deviations are not found in healthy individuals [46]. It has been suggested that lognormal distributions of C_s for circulating tissue enzymes can be explained by the relation:

$$C_s = f_s/FCR$$

where f_s is the steady state release of enzyme per litre of plasma and FCR is the elimination constant. If FCR is normally distributed this relation results in a skewed distribution of C_s [356]. However, biological variation of FCR is 15-20% (SD) for most tissue enzymes (cf. Chapters 6 and 9) and this would produce the same degree of skewness for different enzymes. It must be concluded that variation in steady state release of AST and ALT must be large compared to HBDH.

Another source of error may be introduced by variability of plasma volume. Variation of $V_p(t)$, expressed in ml/kg, is 5-6% in healthy persons and this figure can be reduced by applying corrections for age, sex, heigt, body surface area etc. [529]. Much larger variations in plasma volume may be found in pathological conditions. Moreover, $V_p(t)$ may also show changes in time in various forms of disease. Such changes in plasma volume may be determined in some cases by measurement of changes in hematocrit. An example of this procedure will be given in Chapter 7. In studies with radiolabeled proteins, accurate individual estimates of plasma volume can be obtained by measurement of dilution of injected tracers.

Values of FCR, TER and ERR are usually not known for individual patients. This implies that equation (5.1) is applied by substituting fixed mean values for these parameters. As discussed in Section 3.5, variation betweeen individuals for FCR, TER and ERR (or TER/ERR) for plasma proteins is of the order of 20% (SD). This implies that the last two terms of equation (5.1) may contain substantial error. Little is known about the fluctuations in time of FCR, TER and ERR in one and the same person. Repeatedly injecting CK in the same dog a day-to-day variation in FCR_{CK} of less than 10% was demonstrated, compared to 20% for variation between different animals [517]. The same conclusion can be drawn for CK from Table 5.2. However, it also follows from this table that for AST variation within animals is of the same magnitude as variation between animals.

Table 5.2 Variability in FCR for CK and AST.

	CK					AST				
	D_1	D_2	D_3	D_4	CV (%)		D_1	D_2	D_3	D_4	CV (%)
P_1	0.26	0.37	0.32	0.30	15	P_1	0.23	0.24	0.19	0.21	10
P_2	0.24	0.39	0.31	0.31	20	P_2	0.16	0.21	0.17	0.18	12
P_3	0.26	0.41	0.39	0.30	21	P_3	0.19	0.17	0.19	0.16	8
P_4	0.26	0.37	0.31	0.29	15	P_4	0.32	0.19	0.28	0.23	22
CV (%)	4	5	12	3		CV (%)	31	15	24	16	

Figures indicate values of fractional catabolic rate constants in (hours)$^{-1}$ obtained in 4 different dogs (D_1-D_4) for 4 different homologous enzyme preparations (P_1-P_4). Coefficients of variation are indicated as CV.

From this discussion it follows that error in A(t) as calculated from equation (5.1) is strongly dependent on the time interval of calculations. If A(t) is calculated for a short time t in which extravasation and elimination of protein remains limited, A(t) is mainly determined by the term $V_p(t)C_p(t)$ which can be measured accurately especially if the value of C_s can be individually determined and fluctuations in plasma volume remain limited. For increasing periods of time, however, the contribution of extravasation and elimination becomes more important. Ultimately A(t) is calculated from equation (5.3) and error in A(t) is mainly determined by error in FCR. This situation occurs earlier for rapidly eliminated proteins. An example of the effects of parameter values and the time interval of calculation on error in A(t) will be given in Chapter 6.

5.5 Behaviour of circulating proteins in the dog

In this section it will be discussed how errors as described in the previous sections have affected opinions about the appropriate model for the distribution and turnover of circulating proteins in the dog. This animal was chosen because it has been used in quantitative studies of circulating proteins for more than 40 years.

In 1938 Freeman [163] infused blood from a dog with jaundice into a healthy animal and studied the plasma levels of alkaline phosphatase. It was remarked that the elevated post-transfusion levels returned to normal in a monotonous fashion and at a decreasing rate. Such behaviour would nowadays be described as exponential disappearance and this study probably contains the earliest description of first-order protein elimination. In 1951 this experiment was repeated [113]. On the basis of the textbook value for plasma volume of 50 ml/kg it was concluded that the infused enzyme remained confined to the plasma. Disappearance was "uniformly", i.e. monophasic, with an estimated plasma half-life of 1-2 days. These observations were interpreted as evidence for the absence of loss of intravenously injected proteins to extravascular compartments.

In the same year, however, a different conclusion was drawn from one of the earliest studies with intravenously injected ^{131}I-labeled albumin in the dog [517]. Extravasation of albumin in this study was estimated at 5% of the plasma pool per hour.

In the following years, contradictory results were reported. Some authors mentioned monophasic disappearance of intravenously injected proteins in the dog [455,18], which indicates a single-compartment (plasma volume) model. Others reported biphasic or even tri-phasic disappearance [142,154,512], indicating multi-compartment models. Part of these multi-phasic disappearance curves may have been artefacts caused by injecting mixtures of cytoplasmic and mitochondrial isoenzymes with different elimination rates, but these authors also noticed rapid equilibration between enzyme activities in plasma and lymph. This was considered to prove a relation between the rapid elimination phase of enzyme activity from the plasma and a rapid extravasation of protein to an extravascular pool 2-3 times as large as plasma volume. This latter interpretation does not take into account the small magnitude of lymph flow and the shunt pathway of proteins through the liver sinusoids to the thoracic duct. In these studies lymph samples were obtained from the thoracic duct and, as discussed in Sections 3.2 and 3.3, rapid equilibration between plasma and lymph occurs in the liver and consequently in the thoracic duct. Total lymph flow through the thoracic duct in the dog, however, is 20-30 ml/h [433,153] and it takes 30-50 hours before the total plasma protein pool is transported by this way.

The interest in this field was renewed when studies were made about the relation between the size of a myocardial infarction and plasma levels of cardiac enzymes, again with the dog as test animal. Observed double-exponential elimination of intravenously injected CK was interpreted as rapid extravasation of protein and total distribution space of CK was estimated at 112 ml/kg [424]. These conclusions were soon challenged by authors demonstrating monophasic disappearance of intravenously injected CK in dogs [381,359]. It was concluded that the earlier reported biphasic disappearance was an artefact caused by a CK preparation containing a fraction of damaged but enzymatically still active molecules [381]. Next this was confirmed [382], but contradicted again [440] on the basis of observed biphasic disappearance curves of CK with a rapid initial elimination phase and an estimated transcapillary escape rate of 59% of the plasma pool per hour.

Recently it was demonstrated by means of continuous intravenous infusion of CK and AST, that the bulk of these enzymes remains in the plasma and that the rate of extravasation is slow compared to the rate of elimination [506]. This result was further specified in a report quoting a value of 3% of the plasma pool per hour for the rate of extravasation of ALT [528]. The extravascular pool of ALT was estimated to be 48% of the plasma pool.

The mentioned results can be summarized as follows. After intravenous injection of proteins, a rapid local transcapillary equilibrium is established in the liver and probably also in peripheral lymph. As a result of the limited rate of extravascular transport and the lack of extravascular mixing, this is not an overall rapid equilibration. The overall transcapillary escape rate does not exceed 3-5% per hour for proteins with a molecular weight of more than $M = 40,000$. For rapidly eliminated proteins, as CK ($FCR_{CK} = 0.36$ h^{-1} in the dog; cf. Chapter 9) extravasation is negligible and a one-compartment model can be used. For slowly eliminated proteins, as albumin and ALT, extravasation becomes significant and a multi-compartment model is required.

PART B

Applications

CHAPTER 6

ASSESSMENT OF MYOCARDIAL DAMAGE FROM PLASMA LEVELS

OF CARDIAC ENZYMES

6.1 Introduction

Soon after the discovery of myocardial enzyme release in patients with acute myocardial infarction (AMI) [269], the relationships were studied between maximal levels of aspartate aminotransferase (AST) or latate dehydrogenase (LDH) and histologically assessed infarct size after experimental infarction in dogs [334,399,82]. Although significant correlations were found, these were insufficiently high to allow accurate estimation of infarct size from maximal enzyme levels.

As a result of turnover studies with radiolabeled proteins in the next few years, it became apparent that maximal plasma enzyme levels can only give rough indications of cumulative release of enzymes. More precise estimates require information on the (variability of) elimination rates of enzyme from the plasma and the distribution of enzyme between intra- and extravascular pools. Moreover the relation between maximal plasma enzyme level and the quantity of enzyme released is strongly dependent on the time course of the release process. Sudden release of enzyme results in higher plasma enzyme levels than a more gradual release of the same quantity of enzyme. This development resulted in more sophisticated techniques for the analysis of plasma enzyme levels in patients [530] and in the dog [424]. The latter study demonstrated a high correlation (r = 0.96) between calculated cumulative release into plasma of creatine kinase (CK) and the quantity of CK depleted from the infarcted myocardium. In the years following, quantitative evaluation of enzyme release has been applied in a large number of clinical and experimental studies [299]. Quantitative estimates of myocardial damage obtained with

other methods, based on hemodynamic, electrocardiographic, angio-
cardiographic, scintigraphic and echocardiographic techniques,
were also evaluated by comparison with enzymatic estimates.

Although enzymatic estimation of myocardial damage is now
widely used, a number of experimental findings have caused doubts
about the validity of the underlying concepts. It was pointed out
that estimation of infarct size in gram-equivalents of heart
muscle could be subject to large error if variable fractions of
enzymes are locally degraded and do not reach plasma [384].
Studies in the dog indeed suggest that in large homogeneous
infarctions local degradation of CK may become a dominant factor
(cf. Section 2.6). Other discrepancies have been introduced by
the use of different circulatory models for quantitative description of circulating cardiac enzymes [503; cf. also Section
5.5]. Some of these complications found in experimental studies
do not seem to apply to the clinical situation. Correlations
between mortality after AMI and infarct size [190,345] and between mortality and plasma CK levels [439,244,476] are both
firmly established, so large infarctions in patients obviously do
not release less CK as was observed in the dog. A good correlation was also demonstrated between calculated release of CK and
postmortem determined anatomical infarct size in patients with
AMI [61]. Yet there were also some disturbing clinical results
such as relatively low correlations ($r = 0.70 - 0.80$) between
infarct sizes calculated from different enzymes [532,329,528].

In the present chapter it will be first discussed which features are essential in the circulatory model for the description
of circulating enzymes released from the heart. Physiological
data relevant to this problem have been discussed in Chapter 2. A
technique discussed in Section 4.4, based on simultaneous analysis of plasma time-activity curves of two different enzymes, is
applied in Section 6.3 for the determination of fractional catabolic rate constants for different cardiac enzymes in dogs and in
patients with AMI. Section 6.4 contains an analysis of error in
calculation of cumulative enzyme release. It is shown that this
error is largely determined by the catabolic rate of the enzyme
considered. A rapidly-eliminated enzyme like CK cannot be esti-

mated with the same accuracy as a slowly-eliminated enzyme like
HBDH. Results of the application of various techniques on time-
activity curves obtained from patients with AMI are presented in
Section 6.5. An important question also discussed in this section
concerns the quatitative relation between cumulative release of
cardiac enzymes into plasma and loss of myocardial mass. Results
obtained in patients after open heart surgery are discussed in
Section 6.6. In this case the pattern of enzyme release is complicated by several factors, such as anaesthesia, extra-corporeal
circulation and skeletal muscle damage due to surgery, which
could result in additional release of tissue enzymes.

6.2 A model for the behaviour of circulating cardiac enzymes.

As discussed in Section 2.5, 70-85% of transport of enzymes
from heart to plasma after coronary ligation in dogs, is effected
by direct entry of enzymes into the capillaries. The remaining
fraction of enzyme is transported by lymph but also enters the
bloodstream rapidly though the right lymphatic duct. This implies
that input of enzymes released from the heart may be assumed to
occur intravascularly (cf. Fig. 6.1). Many cardiac enzymes are
rapidly eliminated from plasma and the extravasated quantity of
such enzymes will always be
small compared to the eliminated quantity. The extravascular protein pool $E(t)$ could
in that case be neglected and
a simple one-compartment model
could be used in good approximation [528,506]. Other enzymes, however, are eliminated
more slowly and extravasation
of enzyme may be significant.
For an enzyme like HBDH, with
a fractional catabolic rate
constant of 1.5% per hour, it

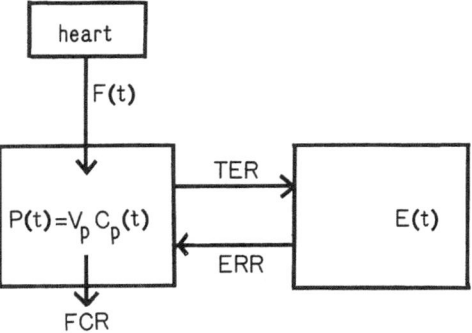

Fig 6.1   Two-compartment model
for circulating car-
diac enzymes.

was shown that extravasation cannot be neglected and a model with at least two compartments has to be used [528].

Values of TER and TER/ERR = $(E/P)_s$ for circulating tissue enzymes in man have only been estimated in a few cases. Infusion of alkaline phosphatase in control subjects resulted in triphasic disappearance from plasma with calculated values of TER = 0.028 h^{-1} and $(E/P)_s$ = 0.70 [95; cf. Table 9.7]. Analysis of simultaneous release of CK and HBDH in patients with AMI resulted in values of TER = 0.014 h^{-1} and $(E/P)_s$ = 0.78 [528]. These values are in reasonable agreement with values obtained for radiolabeled plasma proteins as shown in Chapter 9. Moreover, error in values of TER and $(E/P)_s$ does not necessarily imply a proportional error in calculated cumulative release of enzyme. The process of extravasation is sufficiently slow to keep E(t) small (cf. Fig. 6.1) during the first 10-15 hours after the onset of release. Also, the eliminated quantity of enzyme will always become dominant for long time intervals. This relative insensitivity of calculated cumulative enzyme release to error in values of TER and $(E/P)_s$ will be further demonstrated in Section 6.4. As a consequence, one may use the same fixed mean values for TER and $(E/P)_s$ for different cardiac enzymes. The molecular weights of these enzymes are in the range M = 80,000 - 200,000 and, as discussed in Section 3.3, the blood-lymph barrier shows little discrimination in the passage of macromolecules with molecular weights exceeding M = 50,000.

The model presented in Fig. 6.1 implies first-order intravascular elimination of enzymes. As discussed in section 2.7, it is indeed firmly established that the rate of elimination of circulating cardiac enzymes is proportional to the level of enzyme activity in plasma. If the enzyme is eliminated rapidly enough to make the contribution of extravasation insignificant, first-order elimination results in mono-exponential disappearance from plasma. This was actually observed after experimental injections of homologous CK, AST, LDH, GPI and MDH in the dog, rabbit and baboon [528,506,381,359,496,537,11]. For enzymes which are catabolized more slowly, extravascular elimination of enzyme could become important. However, as discussed in Section 4.2, a model with extravascular elimination of protein - characterized by a fractional catabolic rate constant k_e - is equivalent to a model without extravascular elimination ($k_e = 0$) and parameter values (cf. equation (4.9)):

$$FCR' = FCR + k_e (E/P)_s$$
$$TER' = TER \cdot ERR/(ERR+k_e) \qquad (6.1)$$
$$(E/P)_s' = (E/P)_s \cdot ERR/(ERR+k_e)$$

This implies that in case of extravascular elimination of protein, a model as presented in Fig. 6.1 can still be used if the parameter values are adjusted. From equation (6.1) it is apparent that extravascular elimination of enzymes, if not properly appreciated, results in underestimated values for TER and $(E/P)_s$.

6.3 Estimation of catabolic rate constants for circulating cardiac enzymes

In Chapter 4, the symbol A(t) was introduced to indicate total cumulative release of protein into plasma from time t=0 up to time t. In this chapter we will consider cumulative release of cardiac enzymes per litre of plasma: $Q(t) = A(t)/V_p$. From equation (4.10) one finds for the the model presented in Fig. 6.1:

$$Q(t) = \bar{C}_p(t) + TER \int_0^t \exp(-ERR(t-\tau))\bar{C}_p(\tau)d\tau + FCR \int_0^t \bar{C}_p(\tau)d\tau \qquad (6.2)$$

where $C_p(t) = P(t)/V_p$ is the plasma enzyme concentration (U/l). The bars added to $C_p(t)$ indicate that the enzyme concentration is corrected for the normal steady-state concentration C_s, i.e. $\bar{C}_p(t) = C_p(t) - C_s$. This implies that Q(t) does not include the normal steady-state release of enzyme but only contains the extra release of enzyme due to the infarction at t=0. The second term in equation (6.2) presents the extravasated quantity of enzyme and the last term gives the eliminated quantity of enzyme, both expressed per litre of plasma.

If it is assumed that two different enzymes are released from the heart simultaneously, and in a fixed proportion ρ, we have:

$$Q_2(t) = \rho Q_1(t), \qquad \rho = \text{constant}. \qquad (6.3)$$

As discussed in Section 2.4, there is indeed much evidence for simultaneous release of cytoplasmic cardiac enzymes after myocardial injury. The method discussed hereafter can therefore be applied to such enzymes, but not to a combination of enzymes from different cellular compartments, for instance to a mitochondrial and a cytoplasmic enzyme.

Substituting equation (6.2) into (6.3) one obtains an equation containing the unknown parameters FCR_1, FCR_2, TER_1, TER_2, ERR_1, ERR_2 and ρ. For chosen values of these parameters, the integrals can be numerically evaluated from the observed values $C_{p1}(t)$ and $Cp_2(t)$ for sample times t_j, $j = 1, 2, \ldots n$. The unknown parameter values can in principle be determined by adjustment of the chosen values until the righthand and lefthand side of equation (6.3) become identical. However, this adjustment involves a complicated nonlinear fitting procedure and the number of unknown parameters is too large to expect a well-defined solution.

A first simplification of this problem consists of assuming that $TER_1 = TER_2$ and $ERR_1 = ERR_2$, as discussed in the preceding section. The problem is thus reduced in complexity and can be solved [528] although a considerable uncertainty in obtained parameter values persists. A drastic simplification could be obtained if the rate of elimination of one enzyme, say enzyme no. 1, is considerable higher than the transcapillary escape rate ($FCR_1 \gg TER$) and also much higher than ($FCR_1 \gg FCR_2$). If these conditions would be fulfilled and a relatively short time interval is considered, the contribution of the terms containing FCR_2 and TER could be neglected and equation (6.3) could simply be written:

$$\overline{C}_{p2}(t) = \rho\overline{C}_{p1}(t) + \rho.FCR_1 \int_o^t \overline{C}_{p1}(\tau)d\tau \qquad (6.4)$$

The parameters ρ and $\rho.FCR_1$ could simply be estimated from this equation by use of a standard linear regression procedure minimizing the difference between the righthand and lefthand side of equation (6.4) over all datapoints.

However, equation (6.4) becomes invalid as soon as the eliminated quantity of enzyme no. 2, or the extravasated quantity of one of the enzymes, can no longer be neglected. A better procedure is therefore obtained if the terms containing TER, ERR and FCR_2 are again included in expression (6.3) but are evaluated by using approximate fixed values for these parameters. In this way, the fitting problem can again be solved by a linear two-parameter (ρ, $\rho.FCR_1$) regression procedure. In this case the fitting expression (6.3) only becomes invalid if the values of TER, ERR and FCR_2 in the individual patient would deviate significantly from the fixed values and for long time intervals of fitting.

Validation of this procedure by intravenous infusion of several enzymes in the dog is shown in Table 6.1. Correct mean values of ρ and FCR were obtained. In order to verify whether the variation in obtained parameter values can be explained by the effect of error in the estimation procedures and by biological variation in parameter values, the fitting procedure was also applied to simulated plasma time-activity curves. These simulated curves were obtained by calculation of plasma enzyme activities which would result from a mean release function F(t) and mean parameter values as obtained from fitting. Biological variation in parameter values was simulated by adding a random 20% (SD) variation to these values. Error in determination of plasma enzyme activities was simulated by adding a random 2.5-4.0% error to these calculated activities.

Table 6.2 contains the results of the fitting procedure on plasma enzyme levels measured in patients with AMI. The variability in parameter values, as well as the quality of fit, is in agreement with the values predicted from simulation. An exception is CK(MB) with unexplained variability in ρ and a poor quality of fit. Values of ρ as found for enzyme release after AMI do not deviate significantly from values of ρ as calculated from the cytoplasmic enzyme content of myocardium. For HBDH, CK, GPI and ALT the bulk of enzyme is indeed located in the cytoplasma but for AST this is only true for about 40% of total cellular enzyme activity, while the remaining fraction is contained in the mito-

Table 6.1 <u>Mean parameter values obtained from intravenous infusion of enzymes in dogs with ALT as reference enzyme</u>.

	$\rho \pm$ SD	FCR $\pm$ SD	res $\pm$ SD
AST (n = 12)			
fit over 7 h	1.8 $\pm$ 0.15	0.18 $\pm$ 0.04	3.7 $\pm$ 1.4
simulation	1.8 $\pm$ 0.15	0.18 $\pm$ 0.06	3.3 $\pm$ 0.6
true values	1.7 $\pm$ 0.13	0.20 $\pm$ 0.05	
GPI (n = 12)			
fit over 7 h	0.93 $\pm$ 0.17	0.34 $\pm$ 0.12	5.0 $\pm$ 1.9
simulation	0.90 $\pm$ 0.11	0.40 $\pm$ 0.11	4.5 $\pm$ 1.2
true values	0.86 $\pm$ 0.06	0.36 $\pm$ 0.12	

ρ = infused quantity of ALT/infused quantity of enzyme
FCR = fractional catabolic rate constant (h^{-1})
res = quality of fit, i.e. mean deviation per datapoint(%).

Fixed parameter values used during fitting were: FCR(ALT) = 0.022
h^{-1}; TER = 0.031 h^{-1}; $(E/P)_s$ = 0.48; C_s(ALT) = 29.3 U/l; C_s(AST)
= 12.8 U/l; C_s(GPI) = 66.3 U/l. True values of ρ were obtained
from determination of cytoplasmic enzyme acitvities in the preparation used for infusion. True values of FCR were determined from
bolus injections of the same preparations [528,506].
----
chondria (cf. Table 6.7). As discussed in Section 2.4, only a
small fraction of mitochondrial AST is released after AMI and
this release is much delayed compared to the release of cytoplasmic AST. In Section 6.6 it will be discussed that ρ(HBDH/ALT)
deviates from the value presented in Table 6.2 in the period
following the first 48 hours after AMI. The finding that, after
AMI, enzymes are released in proportion to cytoplasmic enzyme
content of myocardium, can be used to check the crucial assumption of simultaneity of enzyme release. If there would be a
significant time delay in the release of HBDH compared to the
release of either AST, GPI or CK, erroneous values of ρ and FCR
would be found and values of ρ could no longer agree with those

Table 6.2 <u>Mean parameter values obtained from enzyme release in patients with AMI with HBDH as reference enzyme.</u>

	$\rho \pm SD$	FCR $\pm$ SD	res $\pm$ SD
AST (n = 14)			
fit over 48 h	2.45 $\pm$ 0.41	0.093 $\pm$ 0.024	4.2 $\pm$ 2.2
simulation	2.48 $\pm$ 0.45	0.092 $\pm$ 0.029	3.8 $\pm$ 1.0
myocardium	2.28 $\pm$ 0.42 (cytoplasmic AST)		
GPI (n = 14)			
fit over 48 h	0.69 $\pm$ 0.16	0.27 $\pm$ 0.10	4.1 $\pm$ 2.0
simulation	0.75 $\pm$ 0.20	0.24 $\pm$ 0.08	3.8 $\pm$ 0.9
myocardium	0.86 $\pm$ 0.15		
CK (n = 30)			
fit over 48 h	0.12 $\pm$ 0.04	0.20 $\pm$ 0.09	5.5 $\pm$ 2.2
simulation	0.13 $\pm$ 0.03	0.19 $\pm$ 0.07	3.9 $\pm$ 0.9
myocardium	0.14 $\pm$ 0.02		
CK(MB) (n = 16)			
fit over 48 h	1.12 $\pm$ 0.95	0.34 $\pm$ 0.31	8.6 $\pm$ 3.0
simulation	1.24 $\pm$ 0.28	0.30 $\pm$ 0.10	4.8 $\pm$ 0.9
myocardium	0.93 $\pm$ 0.16		
ALT (n = 14)			
fit over 48 h	20.9 $\pm$ 5.4	0.042 $\pm$ 0.019	5.6 $\pm$ 3.0
simulation	21.5 $\pm$ 4.8	0.043 $\pm$ 0.017	4.8 $\pm$ 1.7
myocardium	23.4 $\pm$ 6.9		

ρ, FCR, res : cf. Table 6.1
Fixed parameter values used during fitting were: FCR(HBDH)=0.015 h^{-1}; TER=0.014 h^{-1}; (E/P)$_s$=0.78; C_s(HBDH)=80 U/l; C_s(AST)=8.8 U/l; C_s(GPI)=27.8 U/l; C_s(CK)=47 U/l; C_s(CK-MB)=0 U/l; C_s(ALT)= 7.0 U/l. Values in human myocardium were obtained from biopsies [528]. Myocardial HBDH content was 123 $\pm$ 11 U/g (mean $\pm$ SD).

calculated from heart tissue. This effect is shown in Table 6.3.
Simulated curves were again calculated as described, but the
release function F(t) of AST, GPI and CK was shifted in time with
respect to the release function of HBDH. Comparing the results of
Tables 6.2 and 6.3 it is apparent that no significant deviations
from simultaneity in release of different enzymes can occur.

Comparison of the values of FCR in Table 6.2 with data from
the literature is hampered by a lack of reliable data on the
values of fractional catabolic rate constants of circulating
tissue enzymes in man. Most authors have estimated values of FCR
from plasma disappearance rates of enzymes in patients recovering
from various diseases. In patients with liver damage and rhabdomyolysis values for the apparent exponential diappearance con-

Table 6.3 Effect of non-simultaneous release of enzymes on estimated parameter values.

	AST			GPI			CK		
Δt(h)	ρ	FCR	res	ρ	FCR	res	ρ	FCR	res
+ 4.	4.16	0.045	4.0	1.38	0.13	3.9	0.24	0.11	3.9
+ 2.	3.27	0.062	4.0	1.01	0.17	3.8	0.18	0.14	3.8
+ 1.	2.86	0.073	3.9	0.84	0.21	3.7	0.15	0.17	3.8
+ 0.5	2.67	0.079	3.9	0.76	0.23	3.7	0.14	0.19	3.8
0	2.49	0.086	3.9	0.68	0.25	3.7	0.12	0.20	3.8
- 0.5	2.31	0.094	3.9	0.61	0.28	3.7	0.11	0.23	3.7
- 1.	2.17	0.100	3.7	0.55	0.31	3.6	0.10	0.25	3.6
- 2.	1.80	0.123	3.8	0.40	0.43	3.7	0.077	0.32	3.7
- 4.	1.21	0.186	3.8	0.15	1.00	4.1	0.037	0.64	4.0

Δt = Time shift in hours of enzyme release compared to release of
the reference enzyme HBDH.
ρ ,FCR,res: cf. Table 6.1.
Simulated curves were calculated as described in the text and the
fitting procedure based on the assumption of simultaneous release
was used to estimate values of ρ and FCR. Parameter values used
in the calculation of simulated curves are indicated at Δt=0.

stant k_d of k_d(AST) = 0.041 h^{-1} and k_d(CK) = 0.046 h^{-1} were found [29]. In patients recovering from AMI, values of k_d(CK) = 0.043-0.060 h^{-1}, k_d(HBDH) = 0.013-0.016 h^{-1}, k_d(AST) = 0.06 h^{-1} and k_d(GPI) = 0.17 h^{-1} were observed [532,425,381,329]. As discussed in Section 4.4, however it is inherently impossible to determine FCR in this way because it cannot be ascertained that no further release of enzyme occurs during the disappearance phase. Apparently, the values of FCR have been seriously underestimated, especially for rapidly eliminated enzymes. Reinfusion of plasma taken from patients at the time of maximal enzymes levels was mentioned in two studies. The reported values of k_d(CK) = 0.16 h^{-1}, k_d(HBDH) = 0.015 h^{-1} (n=1) [120] and k_d(CK) = 0.12 $\pm$ 0.015 h^{-1} (mean $\pm$ SE, n = 6) [479] are indeed higher than those usually quoted. For CK these data should be considered cautiously because, as discussed in Section 2.7, this enzyme may be catabolized more slowly after sojourn in plasma.

Little is known about biological variation in values of FCR for circulating tissue enzymes in man, but in the dog this variation is 20-25% for CK, AST, GPI and ALT [506,528,382] and this is of the same magnitude as observed for plasma proteins in man (cf. Section 3.5). Comparison with the variability in obtained values of FCR in Table 6.2 indicates a considerable error of estimation, also apparent from the simulations. Variations of 30-35% in values of FCR are shown, which is consistently higher than the 20% variation in FCR used in constructing the simulated curves. Considering these figures it is apparent that - with the possible exception of AST - use of fixed mean values for FCR will introduce less error in calculated cumulative release of enzyme than use of individually estimated values of FCR. This is also shown in Table 6.4.

6.4 <u>Accuracy in calculation of cumulative enzyme release.</u>

Clinical estimation of enzyme release requires minimal interference with patient care, i.e. a minimal number of blood samples. In this section we show how the accuracy in Q(t) depends on the

Table 6.4 Correlations between release of HBDH and release of
other enzymes during the first 48 hours after AMI.

	AST (n=14)	GPI (n=14)	CK (n=30)	CK(MB) (n=16)	ALT (n=14)
estimated FCR	0.89	0.76	0.61	0.06	0.78
fixed FCR	0.89	0.74	0.81	0.56	0.95

Figures indicate correlation coefficients. Fixed mean values used
for FCR are given in Table 6.2. For HBDH, Q(48) was calculated
by use of the fixed value FCR(HBDH) = 0.015 h^{-1}.

----

sample frequency and the specific features of the enzyme considered, such as values of FCR and C_s.

Equation (6.2) for the calculation of Q(t) can be written as:

$$Q(t) = \bar{C}_p(t) + E(t)/V_p + FCR \int_0^t \bar{C}_p(\tau)d\tau \qquad (6.5)$$

with

$$E(t)/V_p = TER \cdot e^{-ERR \cdot t} \int_0^t e^{ERR \cdot \tau} \bar{C}_p(\tau)d\tau . \qquad (6.6)$$

Using fixed mean values for FCR, TER, ERR and C_s, Q(t) can be
calculated from serial measurement of plasma enzyme concentrations $C_p(t_j)$, j = 1,2,3.....n, i.e. from the time-activity curve.
The integral in expression (6.5) is evaluated by simple numerical
integration, i.e. by calculating the surface area below the
time-activity curve. The integral in expression (6.6) is solved
analytically after linear interpolation of $\bar{C}_p(\tau)$ between the
values found at successive sample times t_j.
    Error in Q(t) as calculated from equation (6.5) may arise from
various sources. The use of fixed mean values for FCR, TER, ERR
(or (E/P_s) and C_s will introduce error due to deviations from

these fixed values in individual patients as a result of biological variation. Values of $C_p(t)$ may contain error due to experimental scatter in enzyme determinations. Also so called discretization errors are introduced by the numerical approximations in the evaluation of the integrals in equations (6.5) and (6.6). The influence of the latter two types of error can be reduced by use of a high sample frequency.

Table 6.5 presents the increase of error in $Q(t)$ due to reduction of the sample frequency. The reference sample scheme contains sufficient samples to make the error due to discretization negligeable. Reduction of the number of samples results in systematic underestimation of $Q(t)$. However, while this systematic deviation can be corrected, the individual variation – shown as the standard deviations in Table 6.5 – represents a true error. Use of sample scheme B, for instance, will introduce errors in $Q(96)$ of 3.9%, 8.0% and 9.3% for respectively HBDH, AST and CK. The small error for HBDH, compared to AST and CK is explained by the fact that the time-activity curve of a slowly eliminated enzyme like HBDH has a more gradual course than for AST and CK (cf. Fig. 6.2).

Table 6.5 Percentage of error in $Q(t)$ due to reduction of sample frequency in 34 patients with AMI.

Enzyme	Sample scheme	$Q(24)\pm SD$	$Q(48)\pm SD$	$Q(72)\pm SD$	$Q(96)\pm SD$
HBDH	A	-2.8±8.4	-1.6±2.5	-1.7±2.5	-0.5±2.2
HBDH	B	-7.0±19	-7.2±4.7	-4.5±3.9	-3.0±3.9
AST	A	-4.3±5.8	-2.2±2.2	-1.2±3.3	-0.0±2.9
AST	B	- 19±19	-15±9.0	-11±8.0	-8.8±8.0
CK	A	-7.5±6.0	-3.6±2.5	-2.3±2.8	-1.1±2.8
CK	B	-31±17	-23±9.9	-17±9.5	-16±9.3

Reference sample scheme: t = 4,8,12,16,20,24,28,32,36,40,44,48, 56,64,72,84,96,108 hours.
Sample scheme A : t = 6,18,30,42,54,78,102 hours.
Sample scheme B : t = 6,30,54,78,102 hours.

Fig. 6.2 presents mean time-activity curves $C_p(t)$ for HBDH, AST and CK, obtained from frequent interpolation and averaging of curves obtained in 34 patients with AMI. Mean cumulative release Q(t), calculated by use of the fixed mean parameter values presented in Table 6.2, is also shown. It is apparent that release of enzymes after AMI continues up to 96 hours after first symptoms but approximately 80% of total release is completed within 48 hours.

Table 6.6 presents error in calculated values of Q(t) due to biological variation in parameter values and scatter in enzyme determinations. The mean functions Q(t) from Fig. 6.2 were used

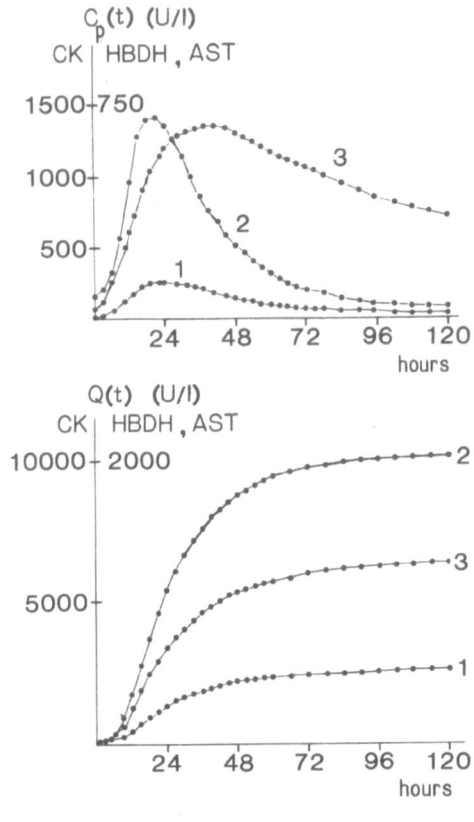

Fig 6.2   Mean time-activity curves $C_p(t)$ and cumulative re-lease Q(t) of AST(1),CK(2) and HBDH(3) in 34 patients after AMI.

to compute time-activity curves which would have occurred in a patient with one parameter value differing a given percentage from the mean value. From the simulated time-activity curve thus obtained, Q(t) was calculated again using mean values for all parameters and the reference sample scheme of Table 6.5. Deviations from the original values of Q(t) are presented.

The effect of error in enzyme determinations was simulated by adding a random error of given magnitude to all calculated values of $C_p(t)$. This procedure was repeated 100 times and Table 6.6

Table 6.6 Error in Q(t) due to biological variation in parameter values and scatter in enzyme determinations.

Δ(%)		HBDH				AST				CK			
time (hours)		24	48	72	96	24	48	72	96	24	48	72	96
	+100	-12	-23	-30	-35	-35	-44	-47	-48	-44	-48	-49	-49
	+ 50	-6	-13	-17	-21	-21	-28	-30	-31	-28	-32	-32	-32
FCR	+ 20	-3	-5	-8	-9	-9	-14	-15	-15	-14	-16	-16	-16
	- 20	3	6	8	11	10	17	21	23	16	22	23	25
	- 50	7	15	23	30	30	56	71	80	53	79	89	94
	+100	-8	-9	-7	-4	-6	-4	-1	1	-4	-2	-0	1
	+ 50	-4	-6	-5	-3	-3	-3	-1	0	-3	-1	-0	1
TER	+ 20	-2	-3	-2	-1	-2	-1	-0	0	-2	-1	-0	1
	- 20	2	3	3	2	1	1	1	1	0	0	0	1
	- 50	5	9	9	7	3	4	3	2	1	1	1	1
	+100	-1	-3	-6	-9	-1	-2	-3	-3	-1	-1	-1	-1
	+ 50	-0	-2	-3	-5	-1	-1	-1	-1	-1	-1	-1	-0
$(E/P)_s$	+ 20	-0	-1	-2	-3	-0	-1	-1	-1	-1	-1	-1	0
	- 20	0	2	3	4	0	1	1	2	-1	0	1	1
	- 50	1	4	8	11	1	2	3	4	-0	1	2	2
	+100	19	16	17	20	9	10	13	16	5	6	9	11
	+ 50	9	8	9	10	5	5	7	8	2	3	4	6
C_s	+ 20	4	3	4	4	2	2	3	4	0	1	2	3
	- 20	-4	-3	-4	-4	-2	-2	-3	-3	-2	-2	-2	-2
	- 50	-9	-8	-9	-10	-5	-5	-7	-8	-4	-4	-4	-5
	± 10	9	7	5	4	6	4	3	3	5	3	3	3
	± 5	5	3	3	2	3	2	2	2	3	2	2	2
C_p	± 2	2	1	1	1	1	1	1	1	1	1	1	1
	0	0	0	0	0	-0	-0	0	0	-1	-0	0	1

Figures indicate error (%) in Q(t) for a deviation of Δ% from a
fixed mean value used in the calculations, or an error of Δ% in
determination of plasma enzyme concentrations C_p (see text).

contains the standard deviation of the distribution of obtained Q(t) values.

The results in Table 6.6 are not much influenced if a reduced sample scheme is used like scheme A or B from Table 6.5. The main effect is that the systematic error in Table 6.5 should be added to the results of Table 6.6.

In order to use Table 6.6, one has to estimate the true magnitude of parameter deviations in patients. As discussed in the preceding section, variations in FCR are probably of the order of 20%. Variations of 20-25% were also demonstrated for TER and $(E/P)_s$ in studies with radiolabeled plasma proteins (cf. Section 3.5). Little is known about the influence of acute myocardial infarction on these values. In studies on the distribution and metabolism of albumin in patients with heart failure, no significant effect on FCR, TER or $(E/P)_s$ was found [415,34]. It was also demonstrated that FCR(CK) is not changed after experimental myocardial infarction in dogs [382]. On the other hand, it was shown that TER is increased in hypertension [348] and increased values of both TER and ERR were found in patients with constrictive pericarditis [351]. In this respect it is important to note that in Table 6.6, as mentioned in Section 6.2, calculated values of Q(t) are rather insensitive to variations in TER or $(E/P)_s$. A 100% increase in TER, for instance, will only cause a 4% underestimation in Q(96) calculated for HBDH. Considering these results, and taking into account that reported variability always contains an error of estimation and therefore overestimates true variability, biological variation in FCR, TER and $(E/P)_s$ may be estimated at 20%.

As discussed in Section 5.4, values of C_s show skewed distributions for most tissue enzymes in man and variability of C_s is less for enzymes with relatively high values of C_s. Use of fixed mean values of C_s, as presented in Table 6.2, will approximately introduce errors between -15% and +30% for C_s(HBDH) and between -20% and +50% for C_s(AST) and C_s(CK) [528,11].

Error in duplicate enzyme determinations is 2-3% for CK and AST and 5% for HBDH. This somewhat larger error in HBDH is caused by a slight degree of hemolysis which may result in some loss of

HBDH from erythrocytes [213].

With these estimates of variability in parameter values and error in enzyme determinations Table 6.5 and 6.6 can be used to estimate the total error in Q(t). As an example we assume that HBDH is sampled according to sample scheme A in Table 6.5. If variations of 20% are taken for FCR, TER, $(E/P)_s$, C_s and an error of 5% is assumed for the assay of HBDH, we

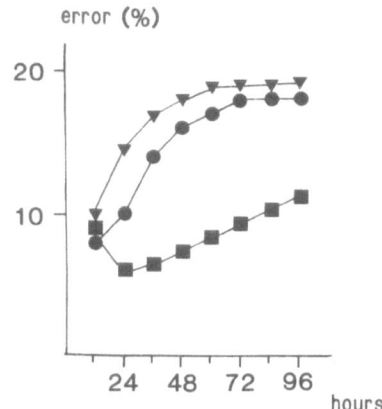

error (%)

Fig 6.3 Mean error in Q(t) for HBDH ($\blacksquare$), AST($\bullet$) and CK($\blacktriangledown$). Sample scheme A from table 6.5 was used.

find from Tables 6.5 and 6.6 that, for independent variations, the mean error in Q(48) can be estimated at:

$$\sqrt{(2.5)^2 + (6)^2 + (3)^2 + (2)^2 + (3)^2 + (3)^2} = 8.6\%$$

Fig. 6.3 demonstrates the mean error in Q(t) thus obtained for t = 24, 48, 72 and 96 hours. Due to the slow elimination of HBDH, a considerable fraction of this enzyme is still present in plasma at the times indicated. This fraction can be measured more accurately than the eliminated fractions of enzyme because error in enzyme determination is small compared to error in FCR. This explains why release of HBDH can be calculated more accurately than release of AST and CK.

In order to calculate total cumulative release of enzyme A(t), values of Q(t) must be multiplicated with the plasma volume V_p. It has been argued that Q(t) is a better clinical index than A(t) because patients with high body weight also have large hearts and large plasma volumes [328]. However, in that case it is assumed that patients with AMI have normal plasma volumes. As will be discussed in Chapter 7, this is not true and considerable changes of plasma volume may occur in such patients. It has been estimated that changes in V_p could introduce errors up to 30% in values of A(t) calculated in patients with AMI [436]. In this study, however, the biphasic response of hematocrit values after AMI, as will be discussed in Section 7.2, was not appreciated and the hematocrit values measured 200 hours after AMI were assumed to present normal values. Consequently, the changes in plasma volume after AMI were overestimated by approximately a factor of 2. Still it follows that the use of a fixed mean value for V_p could introduce errors of up to 15% in absolute estimates of enzyme release and this makes it one of the largest errors to consider. Reduction of this error by use of hematocrit values during the first few days after AMI will be discussed in Section 7.2.

6.5 The extent of myocardial damage in patients with acute myocardial infarction

Fig. 6.4 presents the mean release of CK and HBDH as a function of time in patients with AMI. It is shown that release of enzyme continues up to 96 hours but residual release after 48 hours is relatively insignificant.

An important question to be discussed in this section is whether quantitated release of enzyme after AMI can be related to the loss of myocardium. Several fundamental questions regarding this problem have been discussed in Chapter 2. As shown in Section 2.2,

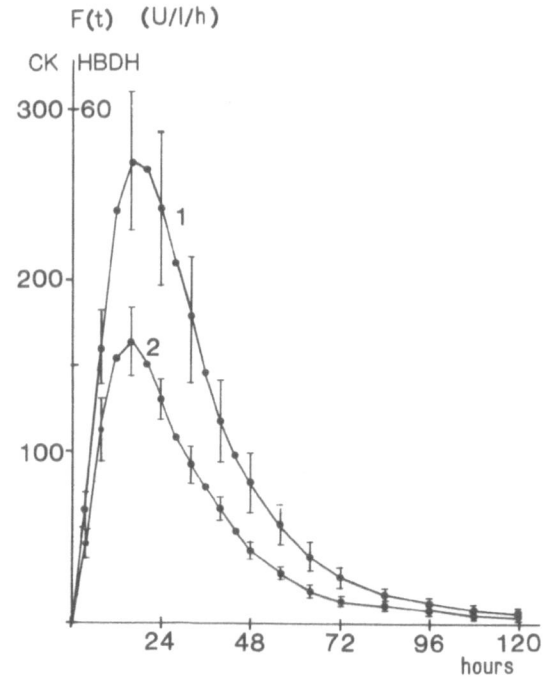

Fig 6.4 Mean release functions F(t) of CK(1) and HBDH(2) in 34 patients after AMI. SEM is indicated.

enzyme content of myocardium, expressed in units per gram of tissue, has a biological variation of 5-10% in most species. This limited variation is of course a first condition for estimation of loss of myocardial mass from plasma enzyme levels in patients. It has also been discussed in Section 2.3, that any appreciable release of cardiac enzymes probably indicates irreversible damage of cardiac muscle cells. This is a second important condition because it eliminates the possibility of a significant loss of enzymes after AMI from cells that remain viable.

The major remaining factor which could obscure the relation between enzyme release and loss of muslce mass, would be the existence of a significant and variable degree of local inactivation of enzymes. Such local inactivation could especially be expected to occur in badly perfused myocardial regions after AMI. As discussed in Section 2.6, a significant local inactivation of CK has indeed been demonstrated after experimental myocardial infarction in the dog, although the relative importance of this phenomenon varies in different studies. In a recent study in the dog [239] a rapid local inactivation of CK was found in ischemic myocardium after coronary ligation, as well as during in vitro incubation of myocardial samples at $37^{\circ}C$. However, in the same experiments, no appreciable local inactivation of LDH could be detected. This stability of LDH was also demonstrated in human hearts. In left ventricular samples from patients who had died without previous history of heart disease, no inactivation of HBDH (i.e. LDH_1 and LDH_2) was found up to 36 hours after death, while CK showed an unpredictable inactivation of as much as 70% of initial activity [203].

A number of studies indicate that local inactivation of enzymes, also including CK, is less important in patients with AMI. As discussed in Section 6.1, it is firmly established that mortality and morbidity due to heart failure after AMI is highly correlated to plasma levels of CK. This has also been demonstrated for AST and LDH [255,89]. This fact contrasts with the finding in the dog that in large experimental infarctions local inactivation of CK becomes so important that actually less CK is released than in smaller infarctions (cf. Section 2.6). Also, a

high correlation (r=0.93) was found in 15 patients between calculated cumulative release of CK and postmortem determined histologic infarct size [61]. In this study, a one-compartment model
with a fixed value of FCR(CK)=0.06 h^{-1} was used and it was assumed that only 15% of the quantity of CK depleted from the heart
was recovered in plasma. Comparison with the value of FCR(CK) in
Table 6.2 shows that the release of CK in this study may have
been underestimated by a factor 3-4. Moreover, as discussed in
Section 2.2, systematic differences between histologic and enzymatic estimates of infarct size must be expected.

A further argument against an important influence of local
inactivation of enzyme follows from Fig. 6.5. Although the group
of patients in this figure only included uncomplicated cases
without manifest cardiac decompensation, the released quantities
of enzyme in the largest
infarctions correspond to
20-25 gram of myocardium
per litre of plasma or,
taking into account a
residual enzyme content
of 20% in the infarcted
tissue and a plasma vol-
ume of 3 litre, a total
infarct size of 75-90
gram of myocardium. Stud-
ies on infarct size de-
termined in patients who
died after AMI [190,345]
have shown that patients
with infarct sizes ex-
ceeding about 100 gram of
tissue invariably died
with signs of cardiac de-
compensation, and this
leaves only a small mar-
gin for local inactiva-
tion of enzyme.

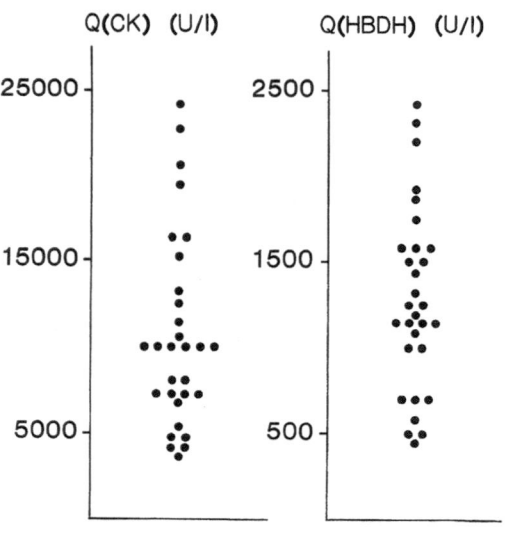

Fig 6.5   Cumulative release of CK
and HBDH during the first
96 hours after AMI. Myocardial content of CK and HBDH
was respectively 865 U/g
and 123 U/g.

Considering the large differences in in vivo and in vitro stability, it should be expected that CK is much more susceptible to
local inactivation than HBDH. This was in fact demonstrated to be
true in the dog [239]. Still it follows from the values of ρ in
Table 6.2 that these enzymes are released into plasma in quantities proportional to enzyme content of myocardium. Again this
fact argues against a large influence of local enzyme inactivation in patients with AMI. A variable degree of local inactivation would also tend to decrease the correlation between calculated release of a labile enzyme like CK and a stable enzyme like
HBDH. Considering the range of observed values of Q(96) for CK
and HBDH, however, an error of 25% in Q(96) for CK and of 10% for
HBDH (cf. Fig. 6.3) would result in a correlation coefficient of
the order of r=0.80 which is close to the observed value presented in Table 6.4.

6.6 The extent of myocardial damage in patients after open-heart surgery.

During open-heart surgery with extracorporeal circulation,
myocardial blood flow and function must be temporarily arrested
in order to allow surgical manipulations. A number of measures
are taken in order to minimize the risk of myocardial damage
induced by such interventions. In some patients, however, the
development of perioperative myocardial damage cannot be prevented and an irreversible loss of myocardial function may occur
even though the surgical corrections were performed successfully.
Due to the rapid development of improved surgical techniques
during the last decade, morality after open-heart surgery has
been much reduced [265,196]. This is clearly a field where a
reliable and easy method for quantification of myocardial damage
is of considerable practical importance and attempts at enzymatic
estimation of perioperative cardiac damage were already started
in 1960 [36]. Since then, many studies have been published on the
relation between enzymatic and electrocardiographic, angiographic
or scintigraphic estimates of such damage [427,65,335,6,319,96,
307,97,156,175,108,131,35,386,490,431,81,116]. Several of these

studies also considered the effect of different techniques of myocardial preservation and it is now firmly established that enzymatic estimation of myocardial damage can be an important tool in the evaluation of cardiac surgery.

Still, cardiac injury is more difficult to measure after cardiac surgery than after AMI because the additional interventions involved may cause enzyme release of non-cardiac origin. In the first place enzymes may be released from blood cells which are damaged during extracorporeal circulation. This damage can be induced by several causes such as mechanical disruption of cells, adsorption of blood cells to non-biological surfaces or contact of blood cells with the "priming" solution used as a substitute for plasma in the cardiopulmonary bypass system. In the second place, a considerable release of enzyme may occur during thoracic surgery due to skeletal muscle damage. As will be discussed below, such release evolves more slowly than release from blood cells. The use of anaesthesia could be a third complicating factor. Release of CK from skeletal muscle has been described in volunteers after anaesthesia without surgery [240] but this will probably be a minor effect compared to skeletal muscle trauma induced by surgery. Anaesthesia could however also influence the values of fractional catabolic rate constants of enzymes [382] or cause liver damage.

The relative importance of the mentioned sources of non-cardiac enzyme release can be judged from Table 6.7. As can be seen from the large LDH/HBDH ratios for skeletal muscle and liver, the LDH content of these organs largely consists of the isoenzymes LDH_5 and LDH_4 which are much less effective in the conversion of alpha-hydroxybutyrate than the "heart specific" isoenzymes LDH_1 and LDH_2. As LDH_5 and LDH_4 are much more rapidly eliminated from plasma than LDH_1 and LDH_2, and also because of the slow onset of enzyme release from skeletal muscle and limited release of hepatic enzymes, plasma HBDH levels after cardiac surgery are not much influenced by skeletal muscle or liver damage. This is not true for the release of HBDH activity due to hemolysis. As illustrated by the much smaller LDH/HBDH ratio, which is close to the value for heart, erythrocytes mainly contain LDH_1 and LDH_2.

Table 6.7   Enzyme activities in human tissues possibly affected by cardiac surgery.

	LDH	HBDH	CK	CK(MB)	cAST	ALT
heart	155$\pm$ 8	123$\pm$ 9	856$\pm$10	132$\pm$27	54$\pm$17	5.1$\pm$37
skeletal muscle						
intercostalis	266$\pm$12	69$\pm$11	3110$\pm$10	28$\pm$ 95	33$\pm$10	2.7$\pm$23
pectoralis	138$\pm$33	42$\pm$44	2580$\pm$38	15$\pm$200	29$\pm$39	6.0$\pm$61
diaphragm	113$\pm$18	48$\pm$24	2377$\pm$14	36$\pm$200	34$\pm$16	6.3$\pm$47
liver	94$\pm$25	25$\pm$14	2.6$\pm$34	–	28$\pm$19	38$\pm$11
blood cells						
erythrocytes	16.5$\pm$ 8	11.7$\pm$ 9	1.7$\pm$ 9	–	0.34$\pm$12	
thrombocytes	0.6$\pm$27	0.3$\pm$33	0.01$\pm$33	–	0.01$\pm$14	
leucocytes	6.5$\pm$20	2.6$\pm$15	0.2$\pm$33	–	0.2$\pm$23	

Enzyme assays are described in refs. [213,492] and activities are expressed in units per gram of wet weight for tissues and in units per ml for blood cells. Figures indicate mean $\pm$ CV(%). Data from ref. [213] were used, assuming normal cell counts of 5 x 10^9 cells/ml for erythrocytes, 0.4 x 10^9 cells/ml for thrombocytes and 0.07 x 10^9 cells/ml for leucocytes.

Moreover, hemolysis occurs during extracorporeal circulation and causes early changes in plasma enzyme levels. This effect is corrected by subtracting the release up to the first postoperative sample from the values subseqently calculated for cumulative release.

Release of CK from skeletal muscle is shown in Fig. 6.6. Such release becomes dominant in the period following the first 12 hours after surgery. It should be noted in Figure 6.6 that in the surgery group the extra release of 10-15 gram-equivalents per litre of CK only amounts to 3-5 gram-equivalents per litre of skeletal muscle (cf. Table 6.7).

During the first 12 hours after cardiac surgery, release of enzymes is mainly of cardiac origin. This is apparent from Fig. 6.6 and also follows from Fig. 6.7.

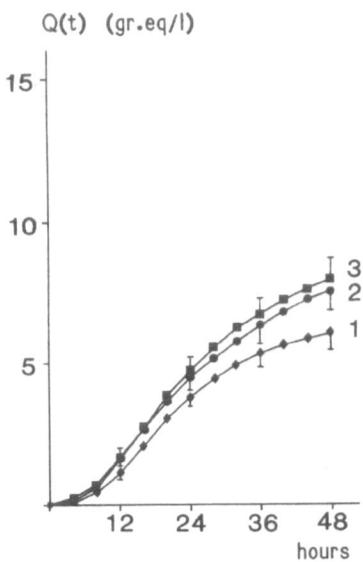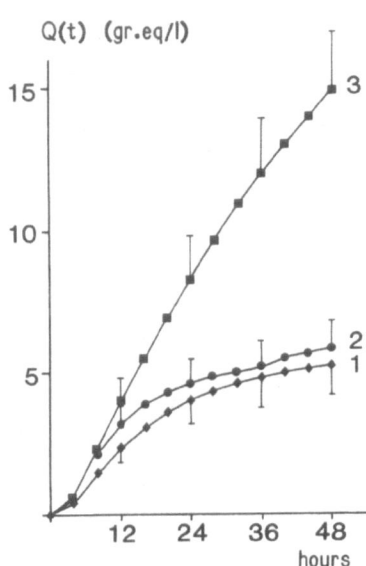

*Fig 6.6   Mean cumulative release of CK(■), HBDH(●) and CK-MB
(◆), expressed in gram-equivalents of heart tissue.
Left panel: after AMI (n=34). Right panel: after
open-heart surgery (n=44).*

The higher correlations for release after cardiac surgery,
compared to release after AMI, are somewhat deceptive (cf. also
Table 6.8) because only a small fraction of total release after
AMI is completed within 12 hours. In contrast, more than 50% of
total enzyme release after cardiac surgery is completed in this
period of time. This fact is also apparent in Table 6.8, where
release of enzyme between 24 and 48 hours in the AMI group still
occurs in proportion to myocardial enzyme content while the
corresponding release in the cardiac surgery group shows large
scatter and is dominated by continuing release of CK from skeletal muscle.

The contribution of liver enzymes to release after AMI and
after cardiac surgery is shown in Fig. 6.8. Although some liver
damage seems apparent in patients with AMI in the period after 48
hours, one gram-equivalent of heart tissue is only 0.13 gram-

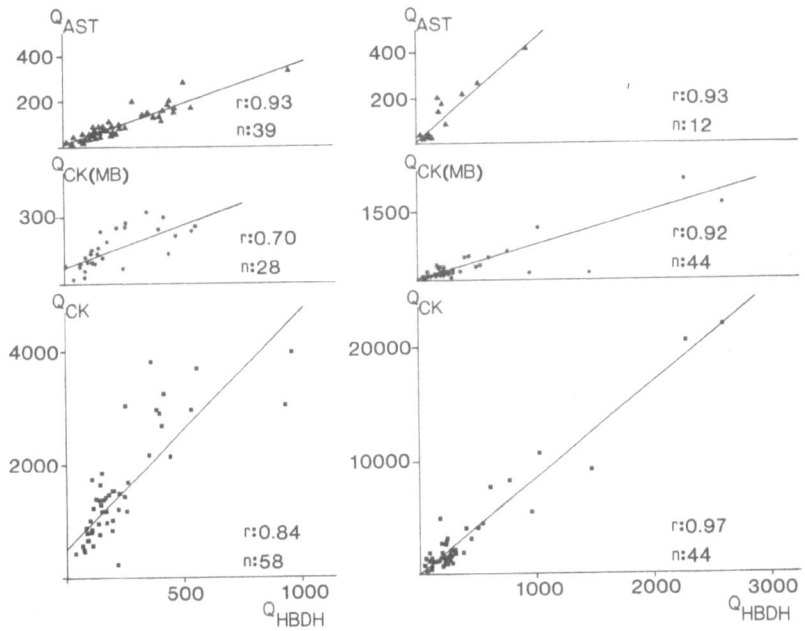

*Fig 6.7 Correlations of cumulative release during the first
12 hours, using HBDH as the reference enzyme.
Lefthand panel: after AMI.
Righthand panel: after open-heart surgery.*

Table 6.8 <u>Ratios of cumulative enzyme release during different
periods of time</u> (mean ± CV%).

	myocardial infarction			cardiac surgery		
time	$\frac{Q-HBDH}{Q-CK}$	$\frac{Q-HBDH}{Q-CK(MB)}$	$\frac{Q-HBDH}{Q-AST}$	$\frac{Q-HBDH}{Q-CK}$	$\frac{Q-HBDH}{Q-CK(MB)}$	$\frac{Q-HBDH}{Q-AST}$
12 h	0.13±13	1.20±42	2.4±31	0.11±53	1.20±52	2.0±52
24 h	0.12±26	0.98±43	2.3±23	0.07±64	1.04±47	2.1±45
36 h	0.12±28	1.04±40	2.3±23	0.05±62	0.95±36	1.9±39
48 h	0.13±33	1.04±37	2.3±18	0.05±66	0.95±32	1.9±42
24-48 h	0.12±36	1.09±41	2.1±26	0.01±150	0.66±87	1.5±78
heart	0.14	0.93	2.3	0.14	0.93	2.3

equivalent of liver tissue for ALT (cf. Table 6.7). Thus, the increase of Q(t) for ALT as shown in Fig. 6.8 indicates a minimal degree of liver damage. Some release of AST from skeletal muscle in the cardiac surgery group is also apparent in Table 6.8 and Fig. 6.8.

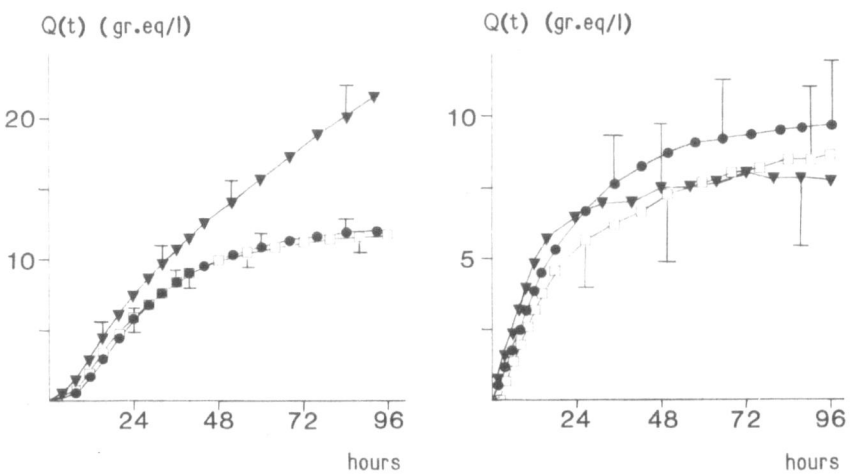

Fig 6.8   Mean cumulative release of HBDH(□), AST(●) and ALT(▼). Left panel: after AMI (n=18). Right panel: after open-heart surgery (n=7)

As discussed in the preceding section, estimates of myocardial damage in patients with AMI can be influenced by changes in plasma volume. Such changes may also occur after cardiac surgery as shown in Fig. 6.9. In fact these changes are strongly dependent on operation procedures and may be much smaller than shown here. Hemodilution as shown in this figure is rapidly compensated and will not

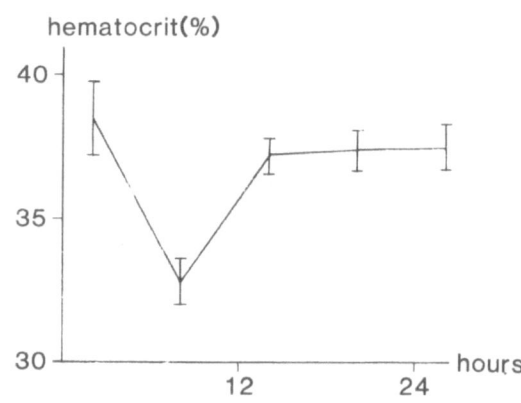

Fig 6.9   Changes in mean hematocrit values in 32 patients after open-heart surgery. (cf. text).

much influence calculated values of Q(t). Still it seems likely
that changes in plasma volume analogous to those observed after
AMI will occur in patients with evolving postoperative myocardial
infarction. Such changes cannot simply be corrected by measure
ment of hematocrits because of
difficulties in obtaining
accurate blood balances in
bleeding patients or in patients receiving blood trans-
fusions. From the results presented in this section it is
apparent that HBDH can be used
for estimation of myocardial
damage after cardiac surgery.
This is however only true if
no excessive hemolysis occurs
during extracorporeal circulation. If elevations of plasma HBDH levels are of the order of a few hundred units per
litre, as may be observed in
unfavourable conditions, large
errors are introduced in calculation of Q(HBDH), especially in case of minor myocardial
injury. It is also apparent
that CK cannot be used because
of skeletal muscle damage
while, to a lesser degree,
this is also true for AST. Use
of CK(MB), although attractive
from the point of view of
heart-specificity, involves
large errors due to its large
fractional catabolic rate constant, as discussed in Section
6.4. An application of the use

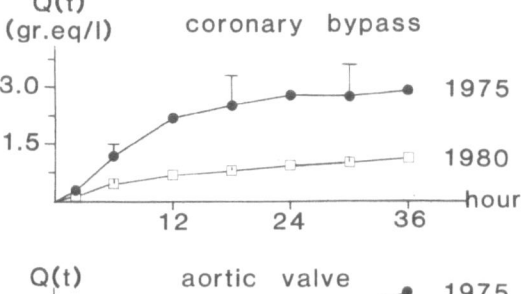

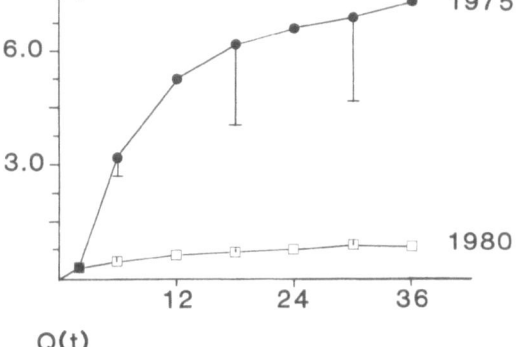

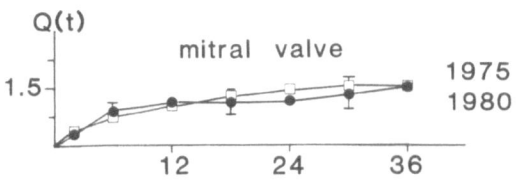

Fig 6.10

Changes during a 5 year period
in cumulative release of HBDH
after coronary bypass grafting
(n=15), aoric valve replacement
(n=10) and mitral valve repla-
cement (n=7). Cf. text.

of HBDH for estimation of perioperative myocardial damage is given in Fig. 6.10. The improvements of surgical techniques in a 5-year period (1975-1980) are shown in this figure. The drastic reduction of myocardial damage in aortic valve replacement was probably associated with a change in myocardial preservation technique. In 1975, continuous coronary perfusion with hypothermic blood was given by selective cannulation of the coronary ostia. In 1980, a potassium-induced hypothermic cardioplegia was used. Examples as presented in Fig. 6.10 demonstrate that assessment of myocardial damage by means of plasma enzyme levels may be usefull even in relatively small groups of patients.

CHAPTER 7

CHANGES IN CIRCULATING MASS OF PLASMA PROTEINS DURING

THE ACUTE PHASE RESPONSE

7.1 Introduction

The concentrations in plasma of several proteins show major changes in response to tissue damage such as caused by surgery, bone fractures or myocardial infarction. This so-called acute phase response consists of a prolonged increase of plasma concentrations for fibrinogen, $alpha_1$-antitrypsin, haptoglobin and $alpha_1$-acid glycoprotein. Moreover, there appears in the plasma a considerable quantity of a protein, called C-reactive protein, which normally is absent or only occurs in trace amounts. Such proteins, defined as trauma-induced liver-produced glycoproteins [262], are called acute phase reactants. The proteinase inhibitor $alpha_2$-macroglobulin has also been described as an acute phase reactant by some authors, but this was denied by others [262].

There may be exceptions to the rule that acute phase reactants are produced in the liver. Endothelium-produced coagulation factor VIII, for instance, also shows increased plasma levels after trauma [373,117,145] and a tissue enzyme like gamma-glutamyl transpeptidase also shows an acute phase-like behaviour [360]. The acute phase reactants as discussed in this chapter are indeed of hepatic origin. This greatly facilitates a quantitative treatment because such proteins are released directly in plasma after synthesis (cf. Section 3.2).

Instead of increased plasma concentrations, several proteins show depressed plasma levels after trauma. This phenomenon is well-documented for albumin and transferrin and these proteins have therefore been called "negative acute phase reactants".

The present chapter will be focussed on the acute phase response after acute myocardial infarction (AMI). The quantitative
treatment of the acute phase response is facilitated by using AMI
as a trigger because the degree of tissue damage can be determined (cf. Chapter 6) and the time at which the trauma occurs is
exactly known. Moreover this aseptic form of tissue damage is not
complicated by the response to infections.

The quantitative treatment as discussed here considers different aspects. Firstly it will be shown that the relatively rapid
plasma volume expansion, which occurs between 3 and 10 days after
AMI, may largly explain the negative acute phase response of
albumin and transferrin. Next it is shown that after a sudden
decrease in the plasma pool of $alpha_2$-macroglobulin in the first
few hours after AMI, the plasma entrance rate has resumed the
normal steady state rate of synthesis within 24 hours. A similar
initial loss is observed for $alpha_1$-antitrypsin. These findings
indicate a rapid proteolysis.

It was suggested already in 1964 that increased synthesis of
acute phase reactants is caused by substances liberated from
damaged or necrotic cells [115]. Shortly afterwards it was demonstrated that inhibition of the production of messenger-RNA by
puromycine or actinomycin D could abolish the acute phase response [321]. Synthesis of C-reactive protein (CPR) could be
demonstrated in periportal hepatocytes within 8 hours after
intramuscular injection of turpentine in rabbits, and after 38
hours CRP was found in most hepatocytes [267]. This finding again
suggests that a mediator, acting initially in the portal hepatic
zones, is responsible for production of CRP by hepathocytes. A
similar mechanism is suggested by the observation that the extent
of the acute phase response after AMI is correlated to myocardial
damage [437,268]. Still, the exact trigger mechanism of the acute
phase response remains to be established.

Assuming that changes in the rates of synthesis of different
acute phase reactants occur simultaneously, the fractional catabolic rate constants can be estimated by comparison of the plasma

curves of these proteins with a reference protein as explained in Sections 4.4 and 6.3. Fibrinogen is especially suited as a reference protein because it shows a pronounced acute phase response while it has well-defined circulatory parameters and a fractional catabolic rate constant which is not dependent on plasma fibrinogen levels (cf. Section 8.3). Using this technique the fractional catabolic rate constants of $alpha_1$-antitrypsin, haptoglobin and $alpha_1$-acid glycoprotein are estimated and compared with values obtained with radiolabeled preparations in the literature. Quantitative estimates of protein synthesis after AMI are presented and compared to the extent of myocardial damage.

7.2 Plasma volume changes in patients with acute myocardial infarction

In 1962 it was shown that the mean hematocrit value in 100 patients with AMI was significantly elevated compared to 100 age-matched control patients [79]. At that time it had been established that the distribution space of erythrocytes is a valid approximation of blood volume. If plasma volume is estimated from dilution of labeled erythrocytes and hematocrit values in blood samples taken from peripheral vessels, a correction factor of 0.92 must be used to estimate the average body hematocrit value from the peripheral vessel hematocrit [49]. If the hematocrit is determined from (micro)centrifugation of blood samples, an additional correction factor of 0.94 has to be used in order to account for the plasma trapped between the packed cells [529]. This early finding of increased hematocrit values in patients with AMI was followed by several studies noting either elevated initial levels or a significant fall of hamatocrit values in the post infarction period [107,446,420,13,522,204,266,150,201]. In several of these studies it was verified that the fall of hematocrits corresponds to a plasma volume expansion as measured by radio-iodinated albumin [420,150,201]. It was also shown that these effects were more pronounced in patients with signs of heart failure treated with diuretics. These findings on the behaviour of plasma volume after AMI contrast with findings in

patients with chronic cardiac decompensation. In such patients
significantly enlarged plasma volumes were found and a decrease
of plasma volume was noted in response to therapy [415,227]. The
significance of hematocrit values for monitoring plasma volume
changes, were also demonstrated during experimental pulmonary
edemagenesis [518,225].

Fig. 7.1 shows the changes in average hematocrit values in a
group of 18 patients with AMI as published [436]. The calculated
decrease of hematocrit values due to diagnostic blood sampling in
the first 10 days after AMI was 1.4%, which implies that the
effect of phlebotomy, as stressed in ref. [204], could not explain the observed fall in hematocrit values.

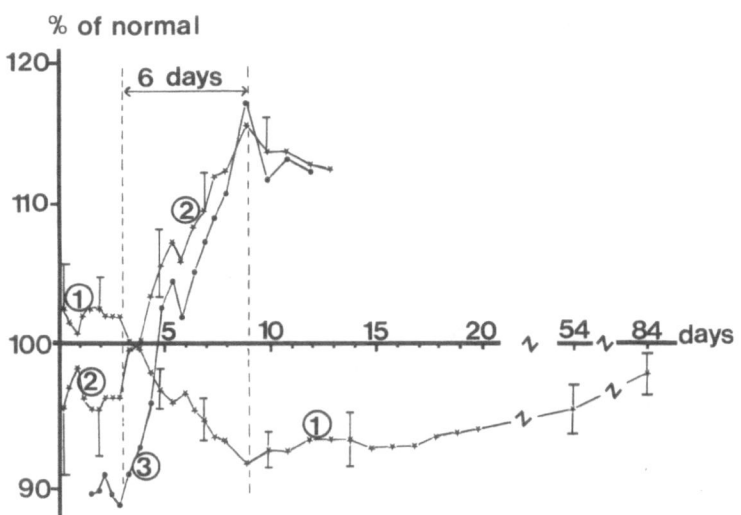

*Fig 7.1   Mean hematocrit values ① in 18 patients after AMI.
Corresponding changes in plasma volume are calculated
for the whole group ② and for 8 patients with pulmonary edema ③ . SEM is indicated.*

Hematocrit values are a relatively insensitive indicator of
changes in plasma volume. If total erythrocyte volume is indicated as VE we have:

$$V_p(t)/VE = (100-H(t))/H(t) = (100/H(t)) - 1$$

where $V_p(t)$ and $H(t)$ are respectively the plasma volume and the hematocrit value at time t. $H(t)$ is expressed as a percentage of blood volume. If it is assumed that VE remains constant during some period of observation, starting at t=0, one has:

$$V_p(t)/V_p(o) = (100/H(t) - 1)/(100/H(o) - 1)$$

which relation can be written as:

$$(V_p(t) - V_p(o))/V_p(o) = -[\frac{100/H(t)}{100/H(t)-1}] (H(t) - H(o))/H(o) \qquad (7.1)$$

Because the factor between square brackets has a value of approximately 2, the relative change in hematocrit is only about one half of the relative change in plasma volume (cf. Fig. 7.1). It has been pointed out that this lack of a one-to-one relation has often caused doubts about the validity of using hematocrit values for monitoring changes in plasma volume [485].

As shown in Fig. 7.1, the mean hematocrit value in patients with AMI is slightly elevated at admission to hospital and this effect is more pronounced in patients with pulmonary edema (cf. also Table 7.1). The most important feature is the rapid fall of hematocrit values between 3 and 9 days after infarction. This period of 6 days is too short to allow any appreciable effect on erythrocyte volume due to changes in erythropoesis. So it can be concluded that a mean plasma volume expansion of 15% has occurred in the whole group, while patients with signs of cardiac decompensation may even show expansions of more than 30%.

Hematocrit values after AMI have a biphasic course. Starting at elevated levels, values fall below normal and subsequent return to normal takes a period of several months. This biphasic response is also apparent from some studies in the literature, for instance ref. [266], but can often not be verified because of the limited periods of observation. Such a prolonged depression of hematocrit values does not necessarily imply a prolonged expansion of plasma volume but could also be caused by decreased synthesis of erythrocytes. Changes in plasma volume in Fig. 7.1 were therefore only calculated for a period of 10 days.

7.3 Plasma volume expansion and the negative acute phase response

Table 7.1 presents the time course of hematocrit values, colloid osmotic pressure, total protein concentration and plasma concentrations of several proteins in patients after AMI. Similar changes in protein concentrations are observed after surgery or after various forms of trauma [522,20]. The well known decrease of plasma levels of albumin and transferrin is also apparent from this table. It will now be verified if this effect can be quantitatively explained by the plasma volume expansion discussed in the preceding section.

The change in time of the total plasma protein pool $P(t)$ is the net result of protein entrance and protein elimination:

$$P(t) = F_e(t) - FCR.P(t)$$

where $F_e(t)$ is the plasma entrance rate at time t. As discussed in Section 3.2, proteins produced in the liver enter directly into plasma. This implies that in normal steady-state circumstances $F_e(t)$ is the rate of synthesis of protein. For non-steady state conditions, $F_e(t)$ is the net effect of synthesis, exchange with the extravascular pool, loss of protein in wound tissue etc. The only term not included in $F_e(t)$ is catabolism of protein with a normal fractional catabolic rate constant FCR. If $F_e(t)$ is expressed as a fraction of the normal steady state rate of protein synthesis $FCR.P_s$, one obtains:

$$F_e(t) = \frac{1}{FCR} \frac{d}{dt} \left(\frac{P(t)}{P_s}\right) + \frac{P(t)}{P_s}$$

$$= \frac{1}{FCR} \frac{d}{dt} \left(\frac{V_p(t)C_p(t)}{V_p(o)C_p(o)}\right) + \frac{V_p(t)C_p(t)}{V_p(o)C_p(o)} \tag{7.2}$$

Table 7.1 Hematocrit, colloid osmotic pressure and plasma protein concentrations in patients after acute myocardial infarction.

time (days)	n total	n pulm. edema	hematocrit (%)		col. osm. pres. (mmHg)	
			total	pulm. edema	total	pulm. edema
0.2	10	6	43.7 ±1.1	44.0 ±1.3	30.1 ±0.5	30.9 ±0.6
1	15	6	43.7 ±0.9	44.9 ±1.3	29.0 ±0.7	30.5 ±1.0
3	18	8	43.3 ±0.7	44.8 ±1.0	27.7 ±0.6	28.7 ±0.9
5	18	8	41.5 ±0.6	42.2 ±1.1	27.9 ±0.6	28.7 ±1.0
7	18	8	40.2 ±0.6	40.3 ±1.0	27.2 ±0.6	27.3 ±1.1
11	15	6	39.4 ±0.7	39.4 ±1.1	26.9 ±0.5	27.9 ±0.4
17	14	6	39.5 ±0.7	39.0 ±1.3	26.8 ±0.4	27.4 ±0.4
54	14	6	40.5 ±0.7	39.7 ±0.8	27.8 ±0.6	27.8 ±0.8
84	14	6	41.5 ±0.6	41.6 ±1.0	27.8 ±0.4	27.7 ±0.9
550	13	6	42.1 ±0.7	42.1 ±1.3	28.3 ±0.6	28.9 ±0.9
controls	18	8	42.4 ±0.7	42.1 ±0.8	27.4 ±0.4	27.4 ±0.4

time (days)	total prot. (g/l)		albumin (g/l)		transferrin (g/l)	
	total	pulm. edema	total	pulm. edema	total	pulm. edema
0.2	70.7±1.4	70.8±2.1	42.9±0.8	41.6±1.0	2.99±0.13	2.93±0.19
1	69.9±1.0	71.3±1.8	41.6±0.6	40.0±0.9	2.85±0.08	2.83±0.15
3	69.8±1.0	69.2±1.3	37.3±1.0	36.1±1.8	2.48±0.06	2.43±0.11
5	68.8±1.0	68.1±1.4	35.6±0.9	34.5±1.7	2.37±0.06	2.32±0.11
7	68.1±1.1	66.6±1.6	35.2±1.0	33.6±1.8	2.40±0.07	2.28±0.12
11	68.9±1.1	68.6±1.2	34.7±1.0	33.8±1.8	2.46±0.07	2.32±0.12
17	69.5±1.1	69.2±0.8	35.9±1.0	34.6±1.8	2.53±0.08	2.38±0.13
54	71.1±1.3	69.7±1.2	39.1±1.2	37.1±2.3	2.58±0.12	2.42±0.12
84	69.5±1.0	69.7±1.5	40.2±1.2	39.5±2.3	2.71±0.10	2.69±0.15
550	72.5±1.3	73.9±2.2	40.1±1.1	39.7±1.2	2.92±0.09	2.77±0.08
controls	70.4±1.1	70.4±1.1	42.3±1.2	42.3±1.2	2.84±0.14	2.84±0.14

Figures indicate mean ± SEM for the total group and for patients with manifest pulmonary edema. Sex- and age-matched control values are also given. Differences in n reflect different times of admission to hospital and death.

Table 7.1 (continued)

time (days)	fibrinogen (g/l)		α_1-antitrypsin (g/l)		α_1-acid glycopr. (g/l)	
	total	pulm. edema	total	pulm. edema	total	pulm. edema
0.2	2.63±0.23	2.85±0.29	2.25±0.10	2.35±0.11	0.78±0.04	0.83±0.05
1	2.98±0.24	3.51±0.37	2.62±0.14	2.88±0.15	0.86±0.04	1.00±0.07
3	5.22±0.36	5.90±0.55	3.62±0.23	4.10±0.39	1.31±0.06	1.47±0.08
5	5.66±0.40	6.40±0.70	3.86±0.28	4.47±0.46	1.50±0.08	1.72±0.10
7	5.51±0.35	6.26±0.59	3.74±0.25	4.17±0.40	1.53±0.09	1.79±0.12
11	4.69±0.37	5.48±0.71	3.33±0.24	3.54±0.44	1.41±0.11	1.69±0.19
17	3.75±0.31	4.13±0.59	2.97±0.21	3.10±0.37	1.21±0.11	1.46±0.18
54	2.65±0.15	2.78±0.28	2.38±0.13	2.50±0.24	0.86±0.05	0.97±0.09
84	2.42±0.07	2.41±0.06	2.21±0.11	2.21±0.21	0.76±0.04	0.82±0.07
550	2.65±0.12	2.58±0.15	2.08±0.10	1.88±0.14	0.71±0.04	0.73±0.05
controls	2.32±0.11	2.32±0.11	2.40±0.08	2.40±0.08	0.64±0.03	0.64±0.03

time (days)	haptoglobin (g/l)		C-reactive pr. (mg/l)		α_2-macroglob. (g/l)	
	total	pulm. edema	total	pulm. edema	total	pulm. edema
0.2	1.49±0.22	1.52±0.25	3 ± 1	5 ± 2	1.85±0.12	1.89±0.17
1	1.67±0.21	1.82±0.31	32 ±10	66 ±16	1.91±0.11	1.87±0.19
3	3.19±0.31	3.53±0.47	38 ±20	208 ±28	1.92±0.11	1.97±0.18
5	3.79±0.34	4.41±0.57	119 ±18	159 ±27	1.82±0.10	1.86±0.14
7	3.80±0.35	4.40±0.59	76 ±12	98 ±16	1.83±0.10	1.87±0.15
11	3.27±0.38	3.71±0.68	35 ± 7	38 ±10	1.79±0.11	1.86±0.23
17	2.73±0.38	3.15±0.64	16 ± 6	18 ±10	1.91±0.12	2.00±0.24
54	1.69±0.21	1.99±0.32	0	0	2.11±0.14	2.16±0.27
84	1.30±0.14	1.51±0.24	0	0	2.08±0.12	2.21±0.23
550	1.60±0.24	1.81±0.39	0	0	2.57±0.17	2.81±0.28
controls	1.67±0.18	1.67±0.18	0	0	2.33±0.13	2.43±0.16

where $V_p(t)$ is the plasma volume and $C_p(t)$ the plasma protein
concentration at time t. Using equation (7.2) $F_e(t)$ can be evaluated from $C_p(t)$ and from control values $C_p(o)$ as presented in
Table 7.1, while the ratio $V_p(t)/V_p(o)$ is calculated from equation (7.1). The mean value for FCR has to be known.

Values of FCR for albumin and transferrin in healthy individuals are well-documented (cf. Chapter 9). Data on these parameters
in pathological conditions are however scarce as discussed in
Section 3.5. For albumin it has been stated that values of FCR
are not much influenced in disease except for gastroenterological
or nephrological disorders [339,515]. After AMI, unchanged values
of FCR were found [415,34]. The effect of plasma albumin levels
on the FCR of albumin, i.e. the deviation of first-order elimination as discussed in Section 3.4, is of little influence as long
as plasma albumin levels do not fall below approximately 75% of
normal [515]. In view of these data, normal steady state values

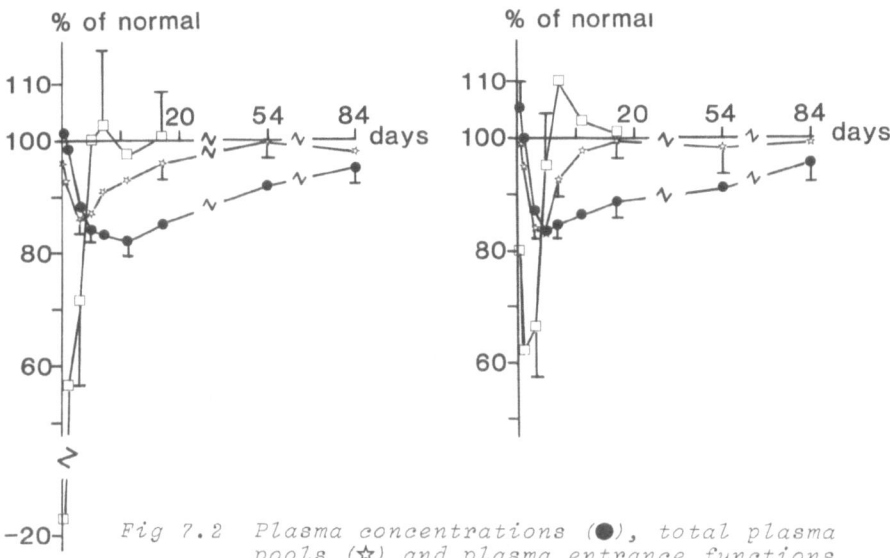

*Fig 7.2 Plasma concentrations (●), total plasma
pools (☆) and plasma entrance functions
(□) in 18 patients after AMI. Left panel:
albumin. Right panel: transferrin.
SEM is indicated.*

of FCR, i.e. FCR(albumin) = 0.0042 h^{-1} and FCR(transferrin) = 0.0072 h^{-1} (cf. Chapter 9) were used in the present calculations.

As shown in Fig. 7.2 there is a considerable reduction in plasma pools of albumin and transferrin during the first 3-4 days after AMI. This reduction is not caused by an overall shift of volume from the intra- to the extravascular pool because plasma volume remains relatively constant during this phase (cf. Fig. 7.1). A possible explanation could be a loss of albumin in the infarcted area. It has been shown that a significant loss of albumin may occur by precipitation of albumin and fibrinogen in wound tissue after surgery [312,118]. A second factor which could contribute to the loss of albumin is the influence of colloid osmotic pressure (COP) on the regulation of albumin synthesis [339]. As shown in Table 7.1 there is a significant elevation of COP during the first 3 days after AMI which could result into reduced synthesis of albumin.

The picture as presented in Fig. 7.2 is consistent with a normal rate of synthesis and a normal rate of elimination of both albumin and transferrin after 5 days. This would imply that during plasma volume expansion, as occurring between the 4th and the 10th day after AMI there would be no net shift of albumin and transferrin from the extravascular pool to plasma. Plasma volume expansion during this period would than be a compensatory mechanism operating in order to keep the total plasma protein concentration constant, in spite of increased synthesis of acute phase reactants. In that case, total protein synthesis is above normal after 4 days, and this would invalidate the hypothesis of re-channeling of aminoacids from albumin synthesis to the synthesis of acute phase reactants during the acute phase response.

In conclusion it is found that the negative acute phase response of albumin and transferrin after AMI is not caused by a prolonged decrease of synthesis but probably is due to a loss of protein and/or depressed synthesis during a few days, followed by a period of plasma volume expansion.

7.4 Consumption of plasma proteinase inhibitors during the early phase after acute myocardial infarction

Complexes between proteinase inhibitors and in vivo activated or released proteinases are eliminated rapidly from plasma, often within minutes [262]. Rapid removal of complexes of plasmin and alpha$_2$-macroglobulin is an example of this phenomenon. Activation of plasminogen by intravenous administration of streptokinase, for example, leads to a significant drop of alpha$_2$-macroglobulin levels in plasma within a few hours after the start of treatment [19,323,457]. As shown in Fig. 7.3, there

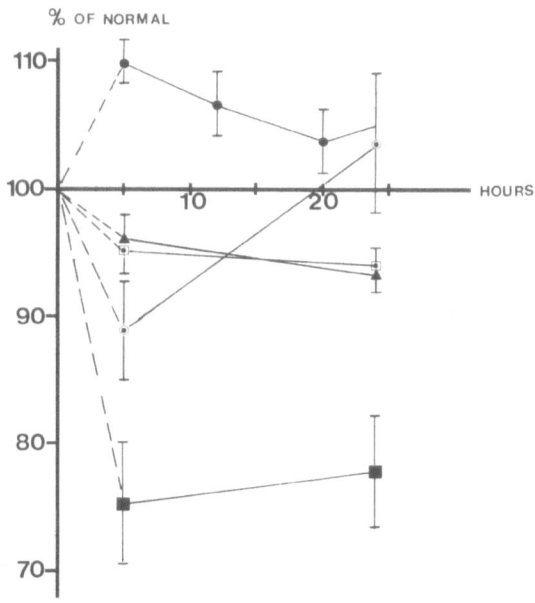

% OF NORMAL

Fig 7.3 *Colloid osmotic pressure (●) and total plasma pools of α$_2$ macroglobulin (■), α$_1$-antitrypsin (◉), albumin (▲) and total protein (◙) in 18 patients after AMI.*

is a decrease in the plasma pool of alpha$_2$-macroglobulin within 5 hours after AMI. The same phenomenon occurs for alpha$_1$-antitrypsin but for this latter protein the effect is obscured by the rapid subsequent increase of plasma levels of this acute phase reactant. The loss of both proteinase-inhibitors is not caused by an overall loss of circulating proteins. As shown in Fig. 7.3, the total plasma protein pool and albumin plasma pool are not significantly changed during the first 5 hours after AMI, as was also found in ref. [266]. Due to the reduction of plasma volume in the early phase after AMI, especially in patients with pulmonary edema, the reduction of the plasma pools of proteinase inhibitors is underestimated when only plasma protein concentrations are considered. Moreover, the effect can only be observed from early observations and comparision with control values, because reduction of $alpha_1$-antitrypsin is followed by a prolonged period of increased synthesis, while for $alpha_2$-macroglobulin the subsequent return to normal is obscured by the plasma volume expansion as discussed in Section 7.2. A fall of plasma $alpha_2$-macroglobulin levels to 78% of normal values was also found in another study of the early phase after AMI [19] but this was not confirmed in a similar study [438].

As shown in Table 7.1 and Fig. 7.3, plasma colloid osmotic pressure (COP) is significantly increased within 5 hours after AMI and returns to normal values within 3 days. This increase in COP in the early phase after AMI, especially in patients with acute pulmonary edema, has been found in several studies [201, 149] and contrasts with earlier work reporting unchanged or even decreased COP in patients with pulmonary edema following AMI]114,449]. Considering the unchanged plasma concentrations of total protein and albumin, this increse in COP might indicate a production of protein degradation fragments due to proteinase activity.

One is tempted to speculate about the effect of increased COP on hematocrit values. Erythrocyte volume is sensitive to plasma COP and changes in hematocrit caused by a 10% change in COP have been described [404], but was also denied [486]. If this effect would have occurred in the data presented in Table 7.1, hematocrit values would have been underestimated during the first 3 days after AMI and the same would be true for the plasma volume expansion as discussed in section 7.2.

The occurrence of proteolysis after AMI, as suggested by Fig. 7.3, is confirmed by studies demonstrating fibrin degradation products in patients after AMI [270,28]. A significant degree of fibrinolysis has also been noted in volunteers after strenous physical exercise [105]

7.5 Calculation of fractional catabolic rate constants from changes in plasma protein concentrations during the acute phase response

From Table 7.1 it is apparent that increases in plasma concentrations of fibrinogen, haptoglobin, $alpha_1$-antitrypsin, $alpha_1$-acid glycoprotein and C-reactive protein after AMI occur roughly parallel. It will now be assumed that the changes in the rates of synthesis of these proteins occur simultaneously. The validity of this assumption will be discussed separately.

The method for estimation of elimination constants as discussed in Section 4.4 may now be applied. This implies calculation of the quantity:

$$\overline{A}(t) = \overline{P}(t) + \overline{E}(t) + FCR. \int_0^t \overline{P}(\tau)d\tau \tag{7.3}$$

with

$\overline{A}(t)$ = $A(t) - A(0)$ = total extra quantity of protein entering the plasma up to time t.

$\overline{P}(t)$ = $P(t) - P(0)$ = increase in the plasma protein pool up to time t

$\overline{E}(t)$ = $E(t) - E(0)$ = $TER._0\int^t \exp(-ERR(T-\tau))P(\tau)d\tau$ = increase in the extravascular protein pool up to time t.

FCR = fractional catabolic rate constant

TER = fractional transcapillary escape rate constant

ERR = fractional extravascular return rate constant.

For parallel release of two different proteins one has:

$$A_2(t) = \rho A_1(t) \qquad \rho = constant \tag{7.4}$$

Substituting equation (7.3) into (7.4) and using fixed mean values for TER, ERR and FCR_2 (of the reference protein no. 2), the remaining parameters ρ and FCR_1 can be estimated from the resulting expression by linear regression. This procedure was described in detail in Section 6.3 and is entirely analogous except for the inclusion of time-variations in the plasma volume. To this end the plasma protein pool $P(t)$ is written as $P(t) = V_p(t)C_p(t)$ and equation (7.4) is divided by $V_p(0)$. The resulting expression can be evaluated from the measured plasma protein concentrations $C_p(t)$ and the ratios $V_p(t)/V_p(0)$, which can be calculated from hematocrit values by use of equation (7.1). Normal steady state plasma concentrations C_s were estimated in each individual patient as the mean of plasma concentrations measured within 8 hours and between 50 to 100 days after AMI. The linear fitting procedure used for the determination of ρ and FCR_1 was performed on the data obtained during the first 20 days after AMI.

Fibrinogen was used as the reference protein, i.e. protein no. 2, in these calculations. As shown in Table 7.1, fibrinogen has a pronounced acute phase response. Moreover, fibrinogen has well-defined circulatory parameters: $FCR = 0.010 \text{ h}^{-1}$; $TER = 0.025 \text{ h}^{-1}$ and $TER/ERR = (E/P)_s = 0.20$, while the value of FCR is not dependent on plasma fibrinogen concentrations (cf. Sections 8.3 and 3.4). It has also been demonstrated that values of FCR, TER and $(E/P)_s$ are not altered in various conditions associated with hyperfibrinogenemia [262].

For alpha$_1$-antitrypsin, haptoglobin, alpha$_1$-acid glycoprotein and C-reactive protein values of $TER = 0.03 \text{ h}^{-1}$ and $(E/P)_s = 1.00$ were used (cf. Chapter 9). In studies on the distribution and turnover of albumin in patients with heart failure, no significant effects on values of TER and (E/P)s were found [34,415] and it seems justified to use fixed mean values for these parameters. The fitting procedure was performed on 14 patients, shown in Table 7.1, who survived a period of 20 days. In this period only 6-8 samples were obtained per patient (cf. Table 7.1) which implies large time-intervals between successive samples and considerable residual deviations per datapoint. Cases in which the mean deviation exceeded 20% were omitted.

Table 7.2 shows the results obtained from this fitting procedure. In order to check these results simulations were performed as described in Section 6.3. Starting from the mean release functions and values of ρ and FCR_1 as obtained, plasma curves were computed for randomly disturbed parameter values (SD=20%). Error in protein determinations (5-10%) was added and the curves were used as if obtained from patients. Comparison of

Table 7.2 <u>Mean parameter values obtained in 14 patients after AMI with fibrinogen as reference protein.</u>

	$\rho \pm$ SD	FCR $\pm$ SD	res $\pm$ SD
α_1-antitrypsin (n=11)			
fit over 480 h	1.3 $\pm$ 0.5	0.017 $\pm$ 0.013	14 $\pm$ 3
simulations	1.3 $\pm$ 0.4	0.019 $\pm$ 0.007	13 $\pm$ 4
α_1-acid glycoprotein (n=11)			
fit over 480 h	3.4 $\pm$ 0.9	0.0098 $\pm$ 0.005	12 $\pm$ 3
simulations	3.4 $\pm$ 0.9	0.0110 $\pm$ 0.005	13 $\pm$ 3
haptoglobin (n=11)			
fit over 480 h	1.0 $\pm$ 0.3	0.012 $\pm$ 0.004	13 $\pm$ 3
simulations	1.0 $\pm$ 0.2	0.013 $\pm$ 0.006	12 $\pm$ 3
C-reactive protein (n=11)			
fit over 480 h	9.6 $\pm$ 9.7	0.24 $\pm$ 0.9	13 $\pm$ 3
simulations	10.0 $\pm$ 3.4	0.62 $\pm$ 2.8	12 $\pm$ 3

ρ = released quantity of fibrinogen/released quantity of the
protein considered
FCR = fractional catabolic rate constant (hours^{-1})
res = quality of fit, i.e. residual percentage of deviation.

Fixed mean values used were: FCR (fibrinogen) = 0.010 h^{-1};
TER(fibrinogen) = 0.025 h^{-1}; TER/ERR(fibrinogen) = 0.20;
TER(other proteins) = 0.030 h^{-1}; TER/ERR(other proteins) = 1.0
Simulations: see text.
----
the parameter values obtained from simulations with the input values in Table 7.2 shows, that values of ρ are correctly esti-mated but values of FCR are slightly biased. Moreover, for C-

reactive protein FCR cannot be estimated from these scarce data
(less than 5 samples were obtained from some patients). Correc-
ting the values of FCR for the bias, the following mean values
are obtained (mean $\pm$ SEM, n=11):

α_1-antitrypsin   : FCR = 0.015 $\pm$ 0.004 h^{-1}
α_1-acid glycoprotein : FCR = 0.0087 $\pm$ 0.0013 h^{-1} (7.5)
haptoglobin   : FCR = 0.011 $\pm$ 0.001 h^{-1}

For alpha$_1$-antitrypsin, this value of FCR is in good agreement
with values obtained from experiments on the turnover of radiolabeled preparations, i.e. FCR = 0.012 - 0.014 h^{-1} (cf. Chapter
9). It has been mentioned [275] that the value of FCR for al-
pha$_1$-antitrypsin does not seem to depend on plasma levels of
this protein. As the results obtained here were found in patients with elevated plasma levels, this finding is confirmed.

For alpha$_1$-acid glycoprotein the values from the literature
are scanty and do not allow proper comparison with the value of
FCR presented in (7.5).

For haptoglobin the value of FCR from (7.5) is somewhat lower
than the value of FCR = 0.015 h^{-1} reported for control patients
(cf. Chapter 9). This could confirm a report on an inverse relationship between the value of FCR and plasma levels of this
protein [161].

It was demonstrated that plasma haptoglobin levels are a
sensitive indicator of hemolysis [333]. As plasma haptoglobin
levels remain in the normal range during the first 5 hours after
the onset of first symptoms (cf. Table 7.1) and because the
subsequent rapid increase of plasma haptoglobin levels is not
delayed compared to the increases in fibrinogen and alpha$_1$-
antitrypsin, it can be concluded that hemolysis is not important
in the acute phase after AMI.

A possible non-simultaneous acute phase response of different
proteins would have an effect on the values of ρ and FCR$_1$ obtained from the fitting procedure. This effect is shown in Table
7.3. As judged from the FCR value for alpha$_1$-antitrypsin, the
time-shift between the response of this protein and fibrinogen

can be maximally 6-12 hours.

Table 7.3 <u>Effect of a time-shift in response of different pro-</u>
<u>teins on estimated parameter values</u>

Δt (h)	α_1-antitrypsin			α_1-acid glycoprotein			haptoglobin		
	ρ	FCR	res	ρ	FCR	res	ρ	FCR	res
+48	1.8	0.012	19	4.3	0.0057	19	1.3	0.008	18
+24	1.7	0.013	16	4.2	0.0061	16	1.3	0.009	15
+12	1.6	0.015	14	4.0	0.0069	15	1.2	0.010	14
+ 6	1.5	0.016	14	3.7	0.0077	14	1.1	0.011	13
0	1.3	0.019	13	3.4	0.0088	13	1.0	0.013	12
- 6	1.2	0.023	13	3.1	0.0103	13	0.9	0.015	13
-12	0.9	0.028	14	2.8	0.0120	14	0.8	0.018	13
-24	0.7	0.047	14	2.1	0.0174	14	0.6	0.028	14
-48	0.2	0.128	14	1.1	-0.034	14	0.3	-0.330	14

Δt = time-shift in hours of protein response compared to the
response of fibrinogen.
ρ, FCR, res: cf. Table 7.2
Simulated curves were computed as described in the text from
release functions shifted in time and parameter values indicated
at Δt=0. The fitting procedure based on simultaneous release
was used to estimate values of ρ and FCR.

Fig. 7.4 shows cumulative release and plasma entrance functions of several acute phase reactants. It is apparent that
stimulation of synthesis during the acute phase response occurs
simultaneous for different proteins. Absolute quantities of al-
pha$_1$-antitrypsin and haptoglobin synthetized during this period
are approximately equal to the extra quantity of fibrinogen
produced, while alpha$_1$-acid glycoprotein is produced at approximately 30% of this rate. As shown in Table 7.2, C-reactive
protein is produced at a rate of about 10% of fibrinogen.

In order to investigate the quantitative relation between myocardial damage after AMI and the acute phase response, infarct size was estimated from myocardial release of HBDH as was described in Chapter 6, but this time corrected for plasma volume changes. Values of Q(96) for HBDH were compared with values of Q(408) for the acute phase reactants, calculated for fixed values of FCR (cf. equation 7.5). For TER and TER/ERR also fixed values were used as given in Table 7.2. The results are shown in Fig. 7.5. A rough, but significant correlation between infarct size and cumulative production of fibrinogen, alpha$_1$-antitrypsin, alpha$_1$-acid glycoprotein and haptoglobin is apparent.

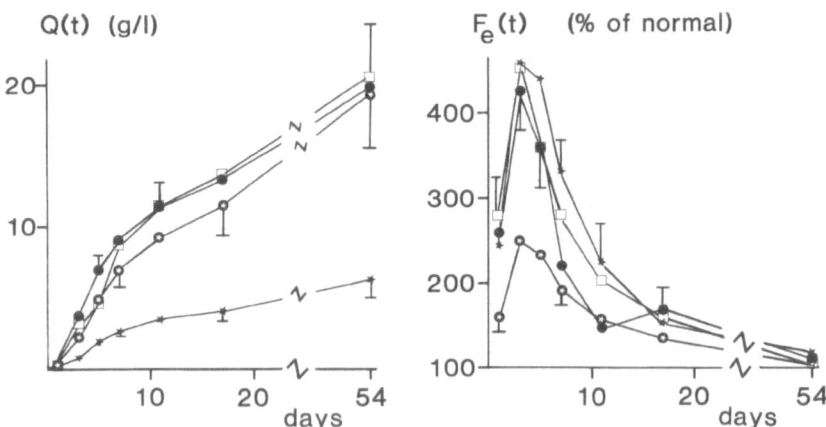

Fig 7.4   Cumulative release Q(t) and plasma entrance function F$_e$(t) of fibrinogen (●), α$_1$-antitrypsin (◉), α$_1$-acid glycoprotein (✫) and haptoglobin (□) in 18 patients after AMI.

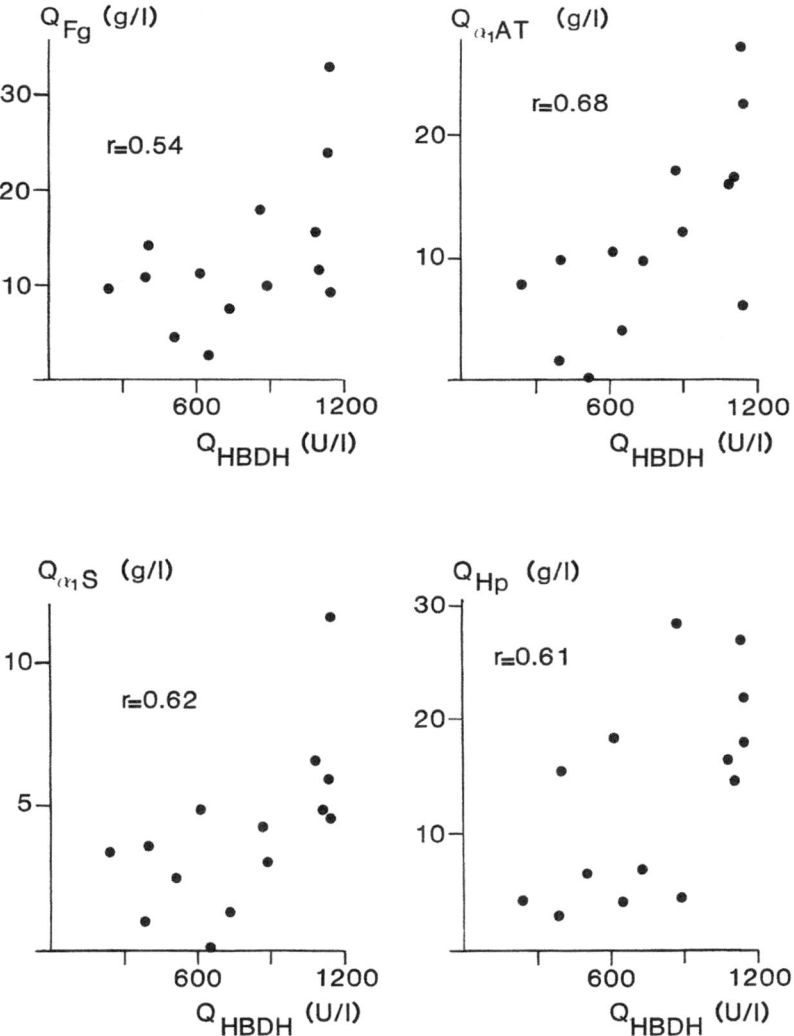

Fig 7.5 Correlations between myocardial release of HBDH in the acute phase after AMI, i.e.Q(96), and excess synthesis of acute phase reactants in the following 3 weeks, i.e. Q(408). Fg =fibrinogen,αAT =α₁-antitrypsin, α₁S =α₁-acid glycoprotein, Hp =haptoglobin.

CHAPTER 8

DOSE-CALCULATION OF BLOOD COAGULATION FACTORS

FOR INFUSION THERAPY

8.1 Introduction

Blood coagulation is a complicated process in which a considerable number of proteins are involved. These proteins are
present in the circulation as precursors of active coagulation
factors. The process of coagulation may be initiated by various
triggers and consists of sequential activation of coagulation
factors resulting in activation of fibrinogen and formation of a
fibrin clot. Most blood coagulation factors have been discovered
due to the existence of inherited protein deficiencies resulting
in a bleeding tendency. Therapeutic infusions of blood or plasma,
containing the missing coagulation factor, have provided early
data on the elimination of circulating proteins. In later years
the physico-chemical techniques for purification and labeling of
proteins were also applied to coagulation factors and today there
is probably no other class of proteins which has been investigated with such variety of techniques (cf. Tables 8.2 and 8.3).

An important result which has emerged from these studies
concerns the crucial property of linearity with respect to protein elimination. Injection of radio-labeled preparations of the
coagulation factors I, II and VIII in healthy controls have
generally provided values for the fractional catabolic rate constant FCR in agreement with values obtained from the disappearance of coagulation factors from the plasma after therapeutic
infusion in patients with deficiencies. As explained in section
5.2, the first procedure measures values of FCR at normal plasma
concentrations, while the second procedure usually measures
values of FCR at plasma concentrations of less than 20% of normal. This agreement of values of FCR proves that these factors

are indeed eliminated by a first-order process. Moreover, it also followed from these results that coagulation factor deficiencies are indeed caused by lack of protein synthesis and not by increased catabolism. Normal values of FCR are also found in bleeding patients and it has been concluded that the loss of coagulation factors in the hemostatic process can be neglected compared to normal catabolism of circulating coagulation factors. Exceptions to this rule are met in severe conditions like extensive bleeding or diffuse intravascular coagulation.

Dose-calculation for therapy in patients with inherited coagulation factor deficiencies presupposes knowledge of the plasma level of coagulation factor needed for effective hemostasis. The choice of a proper level is strongly dependent on the coagulation factor involved and the clinical situation. For some factors, for instance factor XIII, plasma levels of only a few percent of normal are sufficient to stop bleeding in most conditions. Other factors, for instance factor I, may require levels of more than 30% of normal to prevent excessive bleeding after surgery. If the therapeutic plasma level of coagulation factor has been chosen and it has also been decided how long this level must be maintained, the problem is to calculate the quantity of plasma or coagulation factor concentrate needed for the chosen therapy.

Three different situations are frequently met in the treatment of patients with coagulation factor deficiencies. Firstly one may apply a single dose to an ambulatory patient in order to control a non-severe bleeding. In this case one might for instance want to calculate the dose needed to keep the plasma coagulation factor level above 5% of normal for at least 48 hours. A second situation may occur during clinical treatment of a severe bleeding or to control bleeding after surgery. In this case the plasma level of coagulation factor has to be kept above the target level for a longer period of time, say for a period of 10 days. In this situation the problem is to calculate the dose that should be given by continuous infusion or by frequent intermittent infusions. A third situation is met in prophylaxis. In such patients a relatively low plasma level, for instance 5% of normal, is maintained for a long period of time in order to prevent recur-

rent bleeding. As will be discussed in Section 8.4, in this case
one must compromise between infusions of coagulation factors at
long time intervals, in order to limit discomfort to the patient,
and at short time intervals, in order to reduce the quantity of
coagulation factor concentrate needed.

Information needed for dose-calculation in these three different cases are presented in Section 8.4. These data were calculated by using values of catabolic rate constants, extravascular
pool sizes and transcapillary escape rates from the literature,
reviewed in Section 8.3, in a model for circulating coagulation
factors discussed in Section 8.2. A few complicating factors,
such as variable in vivo recovery of infused coagulation factor
preparations, are discussed in Section 8.5.

8.2 A model for the behaviour of circulating coagulation factors

Table 8.1 summarizes the nomenclature of blood coagulation
factors. Missing factors are factor III, factor IV and factor VI.
Factor III, also called "tissue factor" or "thromboplastin" is a
mixtures of protein and phospholipid, obtained from tissue homogenates, which causes rapid coagulation of plasma. Factor IV was
introduced for calcium, indicating that the presence of calcium
ions is crucial in several steps of the sequential activation of
coagulation factors. Factor VI has not been accepted as a separate coagulation factor. Molecular weights in Table 8.1 are taken
from refs. [106,457]. A simplified scheme of coagulation factor
interactions is presented in Fig. 8.1. Activation of coagulation
factors consists of a limited proteolysis, exposing or liberating
the biologically active molecular parts from the inactive precursor molecule. Such activation may start through the so called
"intrinsic" pathway in which factor XII and factor XI are activated in a process involving contact with a foreign surface and
several proteins such as prekallikrein and high-molecular weight
kininogen [457]. A second route of activation is the so-called
"extrinsic" pathway in which factor X is directly activated by
tissue factor in a process involving factor VII and Ca^{++}. A
number of regulatory mechanisms such as activation of factors V,

Table 8.1 <u>Blood coagulation factors</u>

Name	Molecular weight	Traditionally used synonyms
factor I	340,000	fibrinogen
factor II	72,000	prothrombin
factor V	330,000	proaccelerin; labile factor
factor VII	48,000	proconvertin
factor VIII	100,000-2,000,000	antihaemophilic factor A; antihaemophilic globulin (AHG)
factor IX	58,000	antihaemophilic factor B; Christmas factor; plasma thromboplastin component (PTC)
factor X	68,000	Stuart-Prower factor
factor XI	130,000	plasma thromboplastin antecedent (PTA)
factor XII	76,000	Hageman factor; contact factor
factor XIII	320,000	fibrin stabilizing factor (FSF)

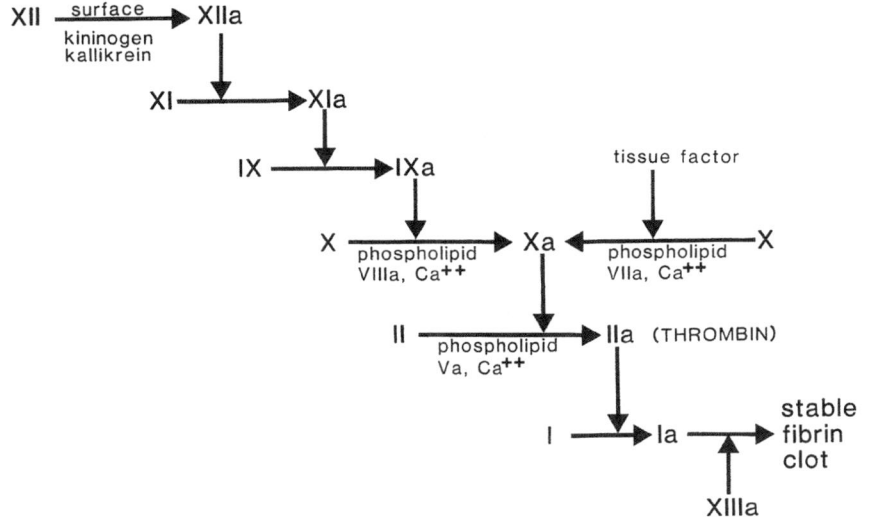

Fig 8.1 Sequential activation of blood coagulation factors

VII and VIII by factor II_a (thrombin), or inactivation of factor II_a by antithrombin III, are omitted in Fig. 8.1. Such positive and negative feedback mechanisms may completely change the picture of activation of coagulation factors. This is also apparent from the observation that a simple sequential activation as shown in Fig. 8.1 cannot account for the severity of clinical sympoms observed in patients with coagulation factor deficiencies. A patient lacking factor XII, for instance, may hardly show any clinical symptoms while the absence of factor IX results in a serious disorder with a need for frequent infusions of factor IX preparations in order to stop bleeding.

With the exception of factor I, normal plasma concentrations of coagulation factors are only approximately known in absolute (mass) values (cf. Table 8.4). Therefore, the plasma content of normal pooled donor plasma is taken as 100% and plasma concentrations are expressed as a percentage of normal. Such concentrations are measured by comparison of the clotting time observed in the plasma with clotting times measured in a series of mixtures of normal plasma progressively diluted with factor-deficient plasma.

A large number of studies using organ transplantation, isolated perfused organs, tissue cultures and immunological techniques have demonstrated that factors I, II, V, VII, IX and X are synthetized in the liver [457,25]. For the factors XII and XIII, direct evidence is lacking but hepatic origin is suggested by the observation that plasma levels of these factors are reduced in patients with liver damage 500,516]. A complicated situation seems to exist with respect to the site of synthesis of factor VIII. Using antibodies against human factor VIII it was shown that this factor is produced in the vascular endothelium and in thrombocytes. However, factor VIII produced in these sites was not biologically active in the coagulation process. Apparently an additional molecular change is needed in order to obtain a fully active form. There are some indications that this change is brought about in the liver or the spleen [63]. As discussed in Section 3.2, hepatic synthesis implies direct intravascular input of protein and this is obviously also true for proteins produced

in the vascular endothelium or released by thrombocytes. The two
main features of the model presented in Fig. 8.2, i.e. intravascular input of protein and first order elimination of protein,
are therefore well-established. Extravascular elimination of
protein is not included in
this model. A study demonstrating that factor VIII is not
detected in the plasma after
intramuscular injection in
patients with haemophilia A
[354], could be an indication
for extravascular elimination
of this protein. In fact this
result would imply that extravascular space behaves as a
sink for factor VIII because
no extravascular return of
protein occurs. This conclusion is however at variance

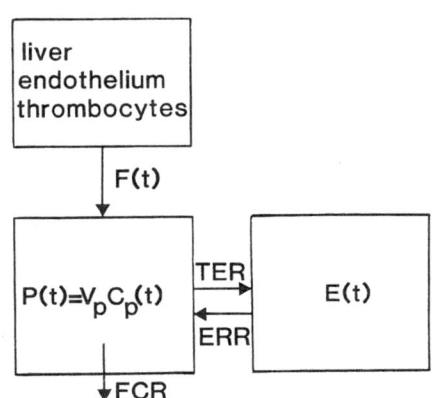

Fig 8.2 *A model for the beha-*
viour of circulating
coagulation factors

with a number of studies (cf. Section 8.3) showing normal biphasic disappearance curves of intravascularly injected factor VIII.
This indicates an extravascular space that can be saturated
whereas an extravascular sink would result in monophasic disappearance with an apparent disappearance rate constant k_d = TER +
FCR. It must be concluded that extravasation of factor VIII in
muscle is of minor importance and this conclusion is supported by
the relative impermeability of skeletal muscle capillaries and
the large size of the factor VIII molecule. Indeed, the biphasic
disappearance curves mentioned indicate a small extravascular
space of about 20% of plasma volume and extravasation of factor
VIII probably is only significant in "leaky" tissues like the
liver and the kidney (cf. Section 3.3).

A similar situation occurs for factor V which is also of large
molecular size and is eliminated sufficiently rapid from plasma
to minimize the effect of extravasation. Also for factor VII,
although much smaller, elimination from plasma occurs so rapidly
that extravascular breakdown of this protein must be of minor

importance. As discussed in Section 3.4 there is much evidence that factor I is eliminated intravascularly although there is no complete concensus on this point.

For the remaining coagulation factors extravascular elimination of protein could occur but, as discussed in Section 4.2, such a situation can still be described with the model presented in Fig. 8.2, except for the following change in parameter values:

$$FCR' = FCR + k_e \cdot TER/(ERR+k_e)$$

$$TER' = TER \cdot ERR/(ERR+k_e) \tag{8.1}$$

$$(E/P)_S' = (E/P)_S \cdot ERR/(ERR+k_e)$$

where FCR and k_e are the fractional catabolic rate constants for respectively the intravascular and the extravascular elimination of protein, and TER and ERR are the fractional rate constants for the transcapillary escape and extravascular return of protein. The variables indicated with accents describe an equivalent model without extravascular elimination ($k_e' = 0$). From these relations it follows that extravascular elimination of protein would result in underestimated values of TER and $(E/P)_S$. This implies that the finding of an exceptionally small extravascular space and a low transcapillary escape rate could indicate partial extravascular elimination of protein. Comparison of the values of TER and $(E/P)_S$ obtained for factors I, VIII and IX (cf. Section 8.3) with the corresponding values of other plasma proteins of comparable molecular sizes (cf. Chapter 9) shows that these values are in the normal range. Extravascular protein pools of about 20% of the plasma pool and transcapillary escape rates of about 2% of the plasma pool per hour are also found for large molecules like alpha$_2$-macroglobulin or immunoglobulin M. Only for factor II, values of TER and $(E/P)_S$ are indeed rather low and this protein might be partly eliminated extravascularly. For factors X, XI, XII, and XIII, available data do not allow separate determination of FCR, TER and $(E/P)_S$ as will be discussed in the next section.

Table 8.2 <u>Experimental procedures used in the study of turnover</u>
<u>and distribution of blood coagulation factors.</u>

A. Intravascular bolus injection of trace amounts of labeled factors in healthy control subjects.
B. In vivo "pulse" labeling by a single injection or oral dose of labeled protein precursors in healthy controls. Incorporation of label is measured in (immuno) precipitates or clots.
C. In vivo labeling by repeated injections, continuous infusions or prolonged intake of labeled precursors.
D. Rapid infusion of coagulation factors in patients with inherited coagulation factor deficiencies.
E. Repeated injections or continuous infusion of coagulation factors in patients with deficiencies.
F. Exchange infusions of a large volume of blood in patients with deficiencies.
G. Measurement of disappearance of coagulation factors from plasma after prolonged therapeutic infusion of these factors.
H. Infusion of high doses of coagulation factor concentrates in healthy controls.
I. Measurement of disappearance of coagulation factors from plasma after pharmacological inhibition of synthesis.
J. Injection of coagulation factor preparations in patients with anitcoagulant-induced deficiencies.
K. Measurement of reappearance of coagulation factors in plasma after termination of anticoagulant therapy or after depletion of the plasma pool.

Table 8.3 <u>Techniques for the analysis of data in studies on cir-</u>
<u>culating coagulation factors (cf. Chapter 4 for de-</u>
<u>tails)</u>

1. Mono- or multi-exponential analysis of disappearance curves of coagulation factors from plasma.
2. Measurement of saturation levels in plasma after prolonged continuous infusion of coagulation factors.
3. Direct estimation of the fractional catabolic rate constant from urinary excretion of labeled degradation products.
4. Direct estimation of the fractional catabolic rate constant from whole-body counting and plasma concentrations.
5. Estimation of the extravascular protein pool at "equilibrium time", i.e. when this pool is maximal.
6. Measurement of the production of labeled protein and the labeled fraction of a low molecular weight substance after administration of labeled precursors.
7. Measurement of the apparent disappearance rate of labeled protein from plasma during the "catabolic phase" after admi-nistration of labeled precursors.

8.3 <u>Estimation of circulatory parameter values for coagulation</u>
<u>factors</u>

As mentioned in Section 8.1, the circulatory behaviour of coagulation factors has been studied in a large variety of situ-ations. Tabels 8.2 and 8.3 summarize the different experimental methods and techniques for the analysis of data used in this field. Table 8.4 presents a selection of the results obtained in these studies as will be discussed below.

Table 8.4   <u>Summary of circulatory parametervalues obtained for</u>
<u>coagulation factors</u>

Factor	C_s (mg/l)	FCR(h^{-1})	TER(h^{-1})	$(E/P)_s$
I	100% = 2000-3600	0.010 ± 10	0.025 ± 40	0.20 ± 25
II	100% = 60 - 170	0.018 ± 20	0.030 ± 50	0.55 ± 25
V	100% = 7 - 13	0.070*	0.025*	0.20*
VII	100% = 0.5 - 0.6	0.40*	0.050*	0.80*
VIII	100% = unknown	0.065 ± 30	0.025	0.20
IX	100% = 4 - 5	0.050 ± 30	0.050 ± 50	0.80 ± 35
X	100% = 7 - 8	0.040*	0.050*	0.80*
XI	100% = 2 - 4	0.020*	0.020*	0.80*
XII	100% = ± 20	0.030*	0.050*	0.80*
XIII	100% = unknown	0.005*	0.025*	0.20*

C_s : normal steady-state concentration in plasma
* uncertain values calculated from few data. Figures indicate
mean values ± CV(%).

Factor I (fibrinogen)

    As shown in Table 8.5, the results obtained in studies on the
turnover and distribution of radio-iodinated fibrinogen are in
good agreement. In order to prevent errors as discussed in Section 5.3, the studies quoted in this table used protein preparations containing less than 1 atom of iodine per molecule of
protein. The results obtained with radio-iodinated protein preparations in Table 8.5 are confirmed by several additional studies, not quoted in the tabel [291,62,102], mentioning values of
k_d = 0.0063-0.0094 h^{-1} in healthy subjects and control patients.
Studies in control patients should be considered critically
because the acute phase character of fibrinogen may result in
prolonged changes in metabolism as discussed in the preceding
chapter. Data obtained from infusion of fibrinogen in deficient
patients are scarce because afibrinogenaemia is very rare. Still
it can be concluded from Table 8.5 that values thus obtained are

Table 8.5 <u>Circulatory parameters obtained for factor I.</u>

Reference and experimental details	Methods (cf. Tables 8.2 and 8.3)	Parameter values ± CV(%) FCR, TER k_d^* in (hours)$^{-1}$	
Takeda '66 autologous ^{125}I-Fg in healthy males	A(1); bi-exponential n = 12 A(3)	V_p=36±10 ml/kg C_s=3.6±14 g/l k_d=0.0086±3	FCR=0.010±7 TER=0.023±56 $(E/P)_s$=0.19±23 FCR=0.010±11
Takeda '78 autologous ^{125}I-Fg in healthy females	A(1); bi-exponential n = 10 A(3)	V_p=36±10 ml/kg C_s=2.8±13 g/l k_d=0.0096±9	FCR=0.011±8 TER=0.029±28 $(E/P)_s$=0.19±14 FCR=0.011±5
Collen '77 homologous ^{131}I-Fg and ^{125}I-Fg in healthy controls	A(1); bi-exponential n = 12	V_p=38±11 ml/kg C_s=2.0±22 g/l k_d=0.0076±10	FCR=0.010±10 TER=0.011±40[**] $(E/P)_s$=0.23±20[**]
Ingram '60 plasma or concentrates	D(1) n = 4	k_d=0.0072±26 (review of different reports)	
Volwiler '55 ^{35}S-cystine	B(7) n = 5	C_s=2.82±4 g/l k_d=0.0013±36	
Brodsky '70 ^{75}Se-methionine	B(7) n = 7	C_s=3.2±28 g/l k_d=0.0037±36	
Stein '78 ^{15}N-glycine and ^{15}N-ammonium	C(6) n = 6	k_d= 0.012±25 (^{15}N-glycine) k_d= 0.018±25 (^{15}N-ammonium)	

[*] k_d is the apparent exponential disappearance constant.
If multi-exponential elimination is observed, k_d is the final
(slowest) disappearance constant.

[**] calculated from the original data.

in general agreement with the values obtained with radiolabeled fibrinogen. As discussed in Section 8.1 this fact indicates first-order elimination of fibrinogen.

The value of k_d for the disappearance of labeled protein from plasma after pulse labeling is much lower than the value obtained for the disappearance of injected radiolabeled protein. This finding has been interpreted as indicating re-utilization of label. It could alternatively be explained by assuming that, after pulse labeling, incorporation of label in fibrinogen may continue for a considerable period of time, for instance due to gradual dilution of the precursor pool. Data obtained from continuous administration of labeled precursors have resulted in values of k_d dependent on the specific precursor used. Apparently these precursor techniques are not yet developed to a point permitting accurate estimates of FCR.

Factor II (prothrombin)

Studies with radiolabeled factor II have shown less consistent results than for factor I, as shown in Table 8.6. The low value of k_d=0.0066 h^{-1}, as found by Benamon-Djiane et al., is in agreement with some studies on the disappearance of this factor in patients with congenital deficiencies. However, values of the order of k_d=0.010 h^{-1} have also been observed in such patients and this latter value was also found after blockade of factor II synthesis with vitamin K antagonists. An even higher value of k_d=0.013 h^{-1} was found by Takeda, using a ^{125}I-labeled factor II preparation. Mean values as presented in Table 8.4 are an average of the results obtained by Shapiro and by Rouvier and correspond to a value of k_d = 0.010 h^{-1}. It is interesting to note that injection of vitamin K after prolonged blockade of factor II synthesis results in a much more rapid reappearance of factor II in plasma than could be explained by the normal rate of synthesis. It seems as if a precursor pool has been formed which can be rapidly converted to factor II. This pool does not consist of the circulating descarboxy-factor II (or PIVKA-II) which appears in the plasma during treatment with vitamin K-antagonists, because

Table 8.6 <u>Circulatory parameters obtained for factor II.</u>

Reference and experimental details	Methods (cf. Tables 8.2 and 8.3)	Parameters values $\pm$ CV(%) FCR, TER, k_d^* expressed in (hours)$^{-1}$	
<u>Shapiro '69</u> homologous ^{131}I-factor II	A(1); bi-exponential n = 7 A(3)	V_p=37.6±5 ml/kg C_s=0.15±13 g/l k_d=0.010±9	FCR=0.018±15 TER=0.037±77[**] $(E/P)_s$=0.62±7 FCR=0.019±12
<u>Takeda '72</u> homologous ^{125}I-factor II	A(1); bi-exponential n = 13 A(3)	V_p=39±4 ml/kg C_s=0.17±17 g/l k_d=0.013±7	FCR=0.027±16 TER=0.063±32 $(E/P)_s$=0.90±22 FCR=0.025±17
<u>Rouvier '75</u> homologous ^{131}I- and ^{125}I-factor II	A(1); bi-exponential n = 16	V_p=39±13 ml/kg C_s=0.13±12 g/l k_d=0.0096±9	FCR=0.017±10 TER=0.018±42 $(E/P)_s$=0.53±23[**]
<u>Benamon '68</u> homol. ^{131}I-fact. II in control patients	A(1); bi-exponential n = 10	k_d=0.0066±22	FCR=0.013±25[**] TER≅0.032(n=2)[**] $(E/P)_s$≅0.84 (n=2)[**]
<u>Soulier '62</u>	D(1)	k_d=0.0056 (concentrate; n=1)	
<u>Biggs '63</u>		k_d=0.0096 (concentrate; n=1)	
<u>Bruning '71</u>		k_d=0.0059 (concentrate; n=1)	
<u>Borchgrevink '59</u>	D(1) I(1)	k_d=0.010 (plasma; n=1) k_d=0.010 (vitamin K antagonist)	
<u>v.d. Meer '68</u> Vitamin K-antagonist	K(1) n = 5	k_d≅0.043 (first 4 hours after intravenous injection of Vitamin K).	

[*]cf. Table 8.5

[**]calculated from the original data

it was shown that the rapid rise of plasma factor II after injection of vitamin K is not accompanied by a simultaneous fall in plasma levels of descarboxy-factor II [276].

Factor V and Factor VII

The turnover of factor V has not yet been investigated by means of labeled preparations and reports on the disappearance of factor V in patients with inherited deficiencies are very scarce. From Table 8.7 it follows that $k_d=0.05$ h^{-1} seems a reasonable estimate for this protein. As no data are available for the calculation of TER and $(E/P)_s$, it is assumed that these values are similar to the corresponding values for factor I, which has the same molecular mass. Using equation (4.6):

$$k_1 + k_2 = FCR + TER + ERR$$

$$k_1 \cdot k_2 = FCR.ERR$$

one obtaines after elimination of k_1:

$$FCR = k_2[1+TER/(ERR-k_2)] = k_2[1+TER/((E/P)_s - k_2))]. \qquad (8.2)$$

Substituting the values $k_2 = k_d = 0.05$ h^{-1}, TER = 0.025 h^{-1} and $(E/P)_s = 0.20$ into equation (8.2) one obtains the value FCR = 0.07 h^{-1} as presented in Table 8.4.

Like factor V, factor VII has not yet been studied by use of radiolabels, but in this case more clinical data are available. Most authors report a rapid initial disappearance phase after infusion of factor VII with a half-life of less than 30 minutes, i.e. much too fast to be explained by extravasation of protein. Apparently, a fraction of the protein is rapidly eliminated from plasma, for instance by adsorption on the endothelium or on blood cells, or by rapid removal in the liver. This latter possibility is suggested by the observation that factor VII can be activated during purification and is rapidly eliminated from plasma after activation.

Table 8.7 <u>Circulatory parameters obtained for factor V and factor</u> <u>VII</u>

Reference and experimental details	Methods (cf. Tables 8.2 and 8.3)	Parameter values ± CV(%) k_d^* expressed in (hours)$^{-1}$
Factor V		
<u>Borchgrevink '61</u> plasma	E(1) n = 6	k_d=0.03-0.06 (repeated infusions in a single patient)
<u>Bowie '67</u> plasma	D(1) n = 1	k_d=0.043

Factor VII		
<u>Hoag '60</u>	D(1); n=7	k_d=0.42±8
concentrate	H(1); n=1	k_d=0.18
<u>Dike '80</u>	D(1); n=6	k_d=0.16±44
<u>Nenci '80</u>	D(1); n=2	k_d=0.44, resp. 0.46
<u>Caen '59</u> concentrate	D(1); n=1	k_d=0.14
<u>Hitzig '58</u>	D(1); n=3	k_d=0.36±18
<u>Hoffman '65</u> blood	F(1); n=1	k_d=0.15
<u>Hjort '61</u>	I(1); n=3	k_d=0.14±5
<u>Frick '58</u> vitamin K-antagonists	I(1); n=4 J(1); n=4	k_d=0.08±5 k_d=0.12±5
<u>Hasselback '60</u>	I(1); n=4	k_d=0.13±5
<u>v.d. Meer '68</u> vitamin K	K(1) n = 5	$k_d \cong$0.030 (first 4 hours after intravenous vit. K injection).

*cf. Table 8.5

From Table 8.7 it follows that pharmacological blockade of synthesis results in a disappearance of factor VII from plasma with a k_d between 0.08 h^{-1} and 0.14 h^{-1}, as demonstrated by several authors. A similar range of k_d has been found after transfusion of factor VII concentrates in patients with inherited factor VII deficiency, but in this case a much more rapid elimination with a k_d of about 0.40 h^{-1} is also found. This discrepancy is rather puzzling because apparently there is a true dichotomy in reported values of k_d and the difference between the two values reported, i.e. k_d = 0.14 h^{-1} and k_d = 0.40 h^{-1}, is too large to be explained by error. The hypothesis that rapid elimination occurs in partially activated preparations does not seem tenable because rapid removal was also observed after infusion of fresh blood (cf. Table 8.7). For the purpose of dose-calculation the highest value of k_d was chosen in order to avoid the risk of insufficient substitution of factor VII.

Reappearance of factor VII following administration of vitamin K, after blockade of synthesis with vitamin K antagonists, initially proceeds at a much slower rate than the normal rate of synthesis. This phenomenon resembles the lag-phase in the disappearance of coagulation factors after a dose of vitamin K antagonists.

Due to the rapid catabolism of factor VII, extravasation of this protein is of minor importance and the apparent disappearance constant k_d approximately equals the fractional catabolic rate constant FCR. Values of TER and $(E/P)_s$ for factor VII in Table 8.4 were taken from the corresponding values for factor IX but these values hardly influence dose calculations for this protein.

Factor VIII

A considerable quantity of data has been accumulated concerning the disappearance from plasma of factor VIII after therapeutic infusion (cf. Table 8.8). A value of $k_d = 0.050 \, h^{-1}$ is consistently found in these studies. Disappearance after such infusion is biphasic although the initial rapid phase is not pronounced and may be absent in some cases. Calculation of TER and $(E/P)_s$ from these data results in values close to the corresponding values for factor I, which seems acceptable for this large molecule. Substitution of $k_2 = k_d = 0.050 \, h^{-1}$, TER = 0.025 h^{-1} and $(E/P)_s = 0.20$ into equation (8.2) yields a value of FCR = $0.067 \, h^{-1}$.

This value of FCR agrees with a value found in a study with radiolabeled factor VIII. In this study ^{125}I-factor VIII was injected in healthy controls and in hemophiliacs, and no significant differences in circulatory parameters were found (cf. Table 8.8). Compared to the disappearance of therapeutic preparations, however, the disappearance of radiolabeled factor VIII did shows a more pronounced rapid phase resulting in higher values for TER and $(E/P)_s$. In fact these values are too high for a large protein and the authors mention the possibility of the presence of a rapidly degraded fraction in their preparation [341]. It is also apparent from Table 8.8 that disappearance of radiolabeled factor VIII after administration of ^{35}S-methionine is much slower than expected. In this study factor VIII was measured by immunological techniques in contrast to the usual measurement of clotting times. Differences in the rate of elimination of factor VIII clotting activity and factor VIII antigen [341] may partly explain these discrepancies, apart from reutilization of label.

Factor IX

Values of k_d after therapeutic infusion of factor IX are in general agreement as shown in table 8.9. In a study on 20 injections, a double-exponential analysis of the plasma disappearance

Table 8.8 <u>Circulatory parameters obtained for factor VIII</u>

Reference and experimental details	Methods (cf. Tables 8.2 and 8.3)	Parameter values ± CV(%). FCR, TER, k_d^* expressed in (hours)$^{-1}$	
<u>Over '78</u> homologous ^{125}I-factor VIII	A(1); bi-exponential n = 6	k_d=0.038±13	FCR=0.059±14[**] TER=0.071±46[**] (E/P)$_s$=0.41±35[**]
same preparation in hemophiliacs	A(1); bi-exponential n = 6	k_d=0.037±50	FCR=0.053±17[**] TER=0.063±55[**] (E/P)$_s$=0.27±56[**]
<u>Green '71</u> homologous ^{131}I-factor VIII	A(1) n = 1	k_d=0.046	
<u>Meyer '67</u> concentrate	D(1); bi-exponential n = 12	k_d=0.050±32	FCR=0.067±32[**] TER=0.030±100[**] (E/P)$_s$=0.22±80[**]
<u>Abilgaard '66</u> concentrate	D(1) n = 16	k_d=0.049±25	
<u>Biggs '63</u> plasma and concentrate	G(1); mono-exponential n = 8	k_d=0.049±38	
<u>McMillan '70</u> concentrate	G(1); mono-exponential n = 26	k_d=0.048±6	
<u>Adelson '63</u> ^{35}S-methionine	B(7); bi-exponential n = 5	k_d=0.011±34	FCR=0.022±34

[*] cf. Table 8.5

[**] calculated from the original data

Table 8.9 <u>Circulatory parameters obtained for factor IX</u>

Reference and experimental details	Methods (cf. Tables 8.2 and 8.3)	Parameter values ± CV(%) FCR, TER, k_d^* expressed in (hours)$^{-1}$
<u>Hoag '69</u> concentrate	D(1); bi- exponential n = 20	FCR=0.048±30[**] TER=0.055±50[**] k_d=0.022±29 $(E/P)_s$=0.79±35[**]
<u>Bowie '67</u> plasma	D(1); bi- exponential n = 2	k_d=0.018 resp. 0.020
<u>Loeliger '67</u> plasma	E(2) n = 3	FCR=0.055±22[**]
<u>Biggs '63</u> concentrate	G(1); mono- exponential n = 3	k_d=0.029±25
<u>Bruning '71</u> concentrate	G(1); mono- exponential n = 2	k_d=0.023 resp. 0.039
<u>Adelson '63</u> ^{35}S-methionine	B(7); bi- exponential n = 5	k_d=0.0033±25
<u>v.d. Meer '68</u> vitamin K	K(1) n = 5	$k_d \cong 0.01$ (first 4 hours after intravenous vitamin K)

[*] cf. Table 8.5

[**] calculated from the original data

curve was given [210]. Using these data, values of TER=0.05 h^{-1} and $(E/P)_s$ = 0.8 are found which are acceptable for a molecule of this size. For FCR a value of 0.048 h^{-1} is found which implies that the true elimination rate of factor IX is approximately twice the apparent disappearance rate from plasma.

Studies on the disappearance of labeled factor IX after administration of ^{35}S-methionine, and on the reappearance of factor IX in plasma after termination of synthesis-blockade, again result in underestimation of FCR as discussed for factor VII and factor VIII.

Factors X, XI, XII and XIII

Data on the disappearance of factor X are scarce but consistent, as shown in table 8.10. In contrast to the situation for factor II, VII and IX, synthesis of factor X is reassumed at a normal rate if treatment with vitamin K-antagonists is terminated by injection of vitamin K.

Factor II, VII, IX and X show physico-chemical similarities which have made it difficult to separate these factor from each other by techniques like electrophoresis, centrifugation or molecular sieving. Considering this fact, one would expect similar values for the transcapillary escape rates and extravascular pool sizes for these molecules. However, a discrepancy exists between the values of TER and $(E/P)_s$ obtained for factor II and factor IX (cf. Table 8.4). As mentioned before, factor II has rather small values for TER and $(E/P)_s$ for a protein of its size. It was therefore arbitrarily assumed that factor X resembles factor IX in this respect. Substitution of the values $k_2 = k_d = 0.02$ h^{-1}, TER = 0.05 h^{-1} and $(E/P)_s$ = 0.8 into equation (8.2) yields a value of FCR = 0.04 h^{-1} for factor X.

The high value of k_d for factor XI quoted by Horowitz seems at variance with the observation that therapeutic infusions of this factor may protect against bleeding for a considerable period of time. The best-documented value for k_d in this case is approximately 0.01 h^{-1}. Factor XI has a molecular weight similar to immunoglobulin G and for this latter protein values of TER = 0.02

Table 8.10 <u>Circulatory parameters obtained for factors X, XI, XII</u>
            <u>and XIII</u>

Reference and experimental details	Method (cf. Tables 8.2 and 8.3)	Parametervalues ±CV(%) k_d^* expressed in (hours)$^{-1}$
Factor X		
<u>Roberts</u> '65	D(1); n=5	k_d=0.022±28 (2 patients)
<u>Bowie</u> '67 plasma	D(1); n=1	k_d=0.020
<u>Caen</u> '59	D(1); n=1	k_d=0.017
<u>Biggs</u> '63 concentrate	D(1); n=1	k_d=0.014
<u>v.d. Meer</u> '68 vitamin K	K(1) n = 5	$k_d \cong 0.025$ (first 4 hours after intravenous vitamin K)
Factor XI		
<u>Rosenthal</u> '65	D(1); n=5	k_d=0.008-0.017
<u>Nossel</u> '64	D(1); n=1	k_d=0.012
<u>Horowitz</u> '65 plasma	D(1); n=2	k_d=0.07
Factor XII		
<u>Josso</u> '64	D(1); n=1	k_d=0.014
<u>Veltkamp</u> '65 plasma	D(1); n=1	k_d=0.013
Factor XIII		
<u>Losowsky</u> '65	D(1); n=2	k_d=0.0041
<u>Britten</u> '67	D(1); n=1	k_d=0.0048
<u>Miloszewski</u> '70 plasma	D(1); n=2	k_d=0.0024

*cf. Table 8.5

h^{-1} and $(E/P)_s$ = 0.8 are relatively well-established (cf. Chapter 9). Inserting these values into equation (8.2) a value of FCR = 0.02 h^{-1} is found for factor XI.

For factor XII, the only two references in the literature quote a value of k_d = 0.014 h^{-1}. Taking the values TER = 0.05 h^{-1} and $(E/P)_s$ = 0.8 from factor IX, which is of similar molecular weight, a value of FCR = 0.03 h^{-1} is calculated from equation (8.2).

Factor XIII is catabolized remarkably slow. Effective hemostasis has been described in patients with factor XIII deficiency using prophylactic infusions of plasma at intervals of 40-90 days [75,306]. Taking the highest reported value for k_d, i.e. k_d = 0.0045 h^{-1}, and values of TER and $(E/P)_s$ of factor I, which is of equal molecular weight, a value of FCR = 0.005 h^{-1} is calculated from equation (8.2).

8.4 Effects of a single dose, intermittent doses and continuous infusion of coagulation factors

In this section it will be discussed which dose of coagulation factor must be infused in order to maintain the plasma concentration of this factor above a chosen level for a given period of time. It will be assumed that the quantity of factor infused in the patient is completely recovered in vivo and this implies that for a number of factors corrections have to be made for partial in vivo recovery. A second assumption to be made is that the fractional catabolic rate constant is in the normal range of values, as discussed in the preceding section. This implies that, although normal biological variation in FCR will be included, no large deviations, such as found in severe hepatic failure or in patients who developed circulating antibodies against coagulation factors, are considered (cf. Section 8.5).

Table 8.11 presents the effects of infusion of a single dose of coagulation factor. These results were calculated for the circulatory model presented in Fig. 8.2 and with parameter values summarized in Table 8.4. Doses as indicated in Table 8.11 must be multiplicated by the required percentage of the plasma coagulation factor level. It is also assumed in Table 8.11 that pre-infusion plasma levels are zero ($C_s=0$). If the patient has only a mild deficiency, for instance a normal steady state level of $C_s=5\%$, this value should simply be subtracted from the chosen target level.

The 95% confidence limits in Table 8.11 were calculated by assuming a biological variation of 20% in FCR, 25% in TER and 20% in $(E/P)_s$. Random deviations of these magnitudes were added to the parameter values and the required dose was again calculated. This procedure was repeated 2000 times and the 95% confidence limits of the distribution of values thus obtained are presented.

Using Table 8.11, one has to estimate the plasma volume of the recipient. In normal adults this volume can be calculated from body weight by use of a value of 40-44 ml/kg. In children a somewhat higher value is found of about 50 ml/kg at the age of 5-15 years and about 55 ml/kg in children less than 5 years old. These estimates can be refined by use of corrections for sex, height, climate, altitude etc. (for instance cf. [529]). However, the error due to use of uncorrected values for plasma volume is small compared to deviations caused by biological variation in FCR (cf. the 95% confidence limits in Table 8.11). An exception must be made for patients after acute bleeding. In such patients plasma volume may be significantly increased [52] and a correction based on determination of hematocrit values may improve the accuracy of dose-calculation.

As an example of the use of Table 8.11 one might consider an ambulatory patient with a severe factor X deficiency (C_s less than 1% of normal), needing therapy for a minor bleeding. It is decided to give a single dose of factor X concentrate which will keep the plasma level in this patient above 5% for at least 48 hours. Total plasma volume in this patient of 70 kg of body weight is estimated at 70 x 0.042 = 2.9 litre. From Table 8.11 it is concluded that the average dose in this case should be 2.9 x 5 x 65.6 = 951 units of factor X, i.e. the factor X content of 951 ml of normal plasma (1 unit is the quantity present in 1 ml of normal plasma). If the therapeutic goal is to be reached with 95% certainty, one should give a dose of 2.9 x 5 x 99 = 1436 units

Table 8.11 Effects of a single dose.

time(h)	Factor I	Factor II	Factor V	Factor VII
2	10.7(10-11)	10.9(10-12)	12.1(11-13)	25.2(19-33)
4	11.3(11-12)	11.9(11-13)	14.6(13-16)	61.9(35-103)
6	11.8(11-13)	12.9(12-14)	17.3(15-20)	145(65-324)
8	12.2(11-13)	13.8(12-15)	20.3(17-25)	308(113-746)
12	13.0(12-14)	15.7(14.18)	27.4(21-37)	878(295-2027)
24	14.9(13-17)	20.9(17-25)	59.3(35-80)	doses too
48	18.2(15-21)	29.3(23-37)	232(91-571)	large to be
72	22.2(18-28)	37.9(27-51)	875(222-3098)	practicable

time(h)	Factor VIII	Factor IX	Factor X	Factor XI
2	11.9(11-13)	12.0(11-13)	11.8(11-13)	10.9(10-11)
4	14.0(13-16)	14.3(13-16)	13.8(12-15)	11.9(11-13)
6	16.3(14-19)	16.8(15-19)	15.9(14-18)	13.0(12-14)
8	18.8(16-23)	19.6(16-23)	18.1(16-21)	14.1(13-16)
12	24.5(19-31)	25.6(20-32)	22.9(18-28)	16.5(14-19)
24	48.3(31-75)	45.3(32-63)	37.4(28-50)	25.1(20-31)
48	161(70-365)	87.5(55-140)	65.6(43-99)	45.6(32-63)
72	522(167-1713)	149(81-277)	103(62-175)	67.3(43-100)

time(h)	Factor XII	Factor XIII
2	11.6(11-12)	10.6(10-11)
4	13.2(12-14)	11.0(10-12)
6	15.0(13-17)	11.4(11-12)
8	16.8(14-19)	11.8(11-13)
12	20.4(17-24)	12.3(11-13)
24	30.8(23-40)	13.3(12-15)
48	48.5(34-66)	14.8(13-16)
72	69.2(46-104)	16.4(14-19)

If a plasma level of x% of
normal is required, the indicated doses should be multiplicated by a factor of x.

Figures indicate doses, in units per litres of plasma, needed to
maintain plasma levels above 1% of normal, i.e. 10 units/l, for
the indicated period of time. The 95% confidence limits are indicated, i.e. the first and the last figure between parenthesis are
sufficient in respectively 5% and 95% of cases.

which would bring the plasma level initially to 1436/2.9 = 495 units per litre or 50% of normal. However, on the average, this latter dose would be sufficient to keep the plasma level above 5% for about 72 hours (cf. Table 8.11). If it is known that the in vivo recovery of activity for the factor X concentrate is approximately 50%, this dose should be doubled. This illustrates that for accurate dose-calculation the in vivo recovery must be documented, preferably for the given patient and the specific preparation used.

Table 8.12 presents the effects of continuous and intermittent infusion of coagulation factors, such as needed for prolonged hemostatic protection after trauma or after surgery. If, in the example just quoted, a surgical intervention is needed and it is decided that the plasma level of factor X should be kept above 30% of normal for a period of 10 days, it follows from Table 8.12 that an initial loading dose of 2.9 x 30 x 16.1 = 1400 units of factor X should be given, followed by continuous infusion of 2.9 x 30 x 0.40 = 35 units of factor X per hour. Alternatively one could give intermittent infusions at intervals of 24 hours. In that case, an initial loading dose of 2.9 x 30 x 34.5 = 3000 units and maintenance doses of 2.9 x 30 x 14.4 = 1250 units are needed. This latter therapy would imply that a larger quantity of factor X is infused than in the case of continuous infusion. This is easily understood because therapy with intermittent doses implies that plasma levels are well above the target level (in this case 30%) for most of the time. Consequently the rate of elimination of factor X from plasma will be higher than during continuous infusion when the plasma level is kept approximately at the target level. In the example given, a dose of 24 x 35 = 840 units per 24 hours is needed for continuous infusion and this implies that intermittent infusions are a factor of 1250/840 = 1.5 more expensive than continuous infusion. This is indicated by the column R in table 8.12.

The reduction in costs by more frequent infusion may be even more pronounced than in this example. For instance, it follows from Table 8.12 that injection of factor VIII at 12 hour intervals implies a reduction by a factor 3 compared to the quantity

Table 8.12 Effects of continuous infusion and repeated doses.

Δt (h)	D_O	Factor I D	R	D_O	Factor II D	R
0	10.6(9.7-12)	0.10(0.07-0.13)	1.0	13.6(11-17)	0.17(0.11-0.22)	1.0
2	10.8(9.9-12)	0.20(0.13-0.27)	1.0	14.1(12-17)	0.35(0.23-0.46)	1.0
4	11.0(10-12)	0.41(0.28-0.55)	1.0	14.5(12-18)	0.70(0.47-0.95)	1.0
6	11.2(10-12)	0.62(0.42-0.83)	1.0	15.0(12-18)	1.07(0.67-1.4)	1.1
8	11.5(11-13)	0.83(0.55-1.1)	1.0	15.5(12-19)	1.45(0.94-2.0)	1.1
12	11.9(11-13)	1.27(0.84-1.7)	1.1	16.5(14-20)	2.25(1.4-3.1)	1.1
24	13.4(12-15)	2.68(1.7-3.7)	1.1	19.5(16-24)	4.90(3.0-7.0)	1.2
48	16.7(14-19)	5.96(3.7-8.5)	1.2	26.4(21-33)	11.4(6.9-17)	1.3
72	20.7(16-26)	9.95(5.9-15)	1.4	34.7(25-47)	19.7(11-31)	1.4

Δt (h)	D_O	Factor V D	R	D_O	Factor VII D	R
0	9.7(9.1-11)	0.75(0.50-1.0)	1.0	9.0(9-12)	4.20(2.8-5.6)	1.0
2	11.4(11-13)	1.62(1.1-2.2)	1.1	25.2(19-47)	13.0(7.8-20)	1.6
4	13.5(12-15)	3.49(2.3-4.9)	1.2	85.6(39-181)	41.4(19-74)	2.4
6	15.8(13-18)	5.65(3.5-8.1)	1.3	213(78-525)	96.8(40-211)	3.8
8	18.4(15-22)	8.12(5.1-12)	1.4	404(133-961)	190(72-424)	5.6
12	24.7(19-33)	14.0(8.4-22)	1.6	869(306-1941)	476(176-1042)	9.1
24	55.1(32-92)	44.0(22-81)	2.4	doses too large to be practicable		
48	227(88-563)	216(77-552)	5.9			
72	870(218-3087)	858(208-3075)	17			

Figures indicate doses in units per litre of plasma and 95% confidence limits as in Table 8.11.

Δt = time interval between successive doses;
D_O = loading dose;
D = maintenance dose;
R = ratio of quantities needed (see text).
Values for continuous infusion are entered at $\Delta t=0$ and in this case D indicates the quantity infused per hour.

Table 8.12 (continued)

Δt (h)	D_0	Factor VIII D	R	Factor IX D	D_0	R
0	9.8(9.2–11)	0.65(0.43–0.86)	1.0	0.50(0.34–0.67)	16.0(12–22)	1.0
2	11.3(10–12)	1.39(0.91–1.9)	1.1	1.05(0.68–1.4)	17.7(13–24)	1.1
4	13.0(12–15)	2.96(1.9–4.2)	1.1	2.21(1.4–3.0)	19.4(14–26)	1.1
6	14.9(13–17)	4.74(2.9–6.6)	1.2	3.47(2.2–4.9)	21.2(15–28)	1.2
8	17.0(14–20)	6.75(4.2–9.8)	1.3	4.85(3.0–6.9)	23.1(17–31)	1.2
12	22.0(17–28)	11.5(6.8–18)	1.5	7.95(4.8–12)	27.2(20–37)	1.3
24	44.6(28–70)	33.7(17–58)	2.2	20.0(11–31)	41.6(29–59)	1.7
48	157(67–358)	146(55–345)	4.8	56.9(29–103)	80.1(50–129)	2.4
72	517(163–1709)	506(150–1699)	11	118(54–242)	141(76–266)	3.2

Δt (h)	D_0	Factor X D	R	Factor XI D	D_0	R
0	16.1(12–21)	0.40(0.27–0.53)	1.0	0.25(0.17–0.33)	16.0(11–22)	1.0
2	17.4(13–23)	0.83(0.54–1.1)	1.0	0.51(0.34–0.69)	16.8(12–23)	1.0
4	18.7(14–25)	1.73(1.1–2.3)	1.1	1.05(0.69–1.4)	17.6(13–24)	1.1
6	20.1(15–26)	2.70(1.7–3.8)	1.1	1.62(1.1–2.2)	18.5(14–26)	1.1
8	21.5(16–28)	3.73(2.4–5.3)	1.2	2.21(1.5–3.1)	19.4(14–26)	1.1
12	24.5(18–32)	6.00(3.8–8.6)	1.3	3.48(2.2–4.9)	21.2(15–29)	1.2
24	34.5(25–46)	14.4(8.6–23)	1.5	8.00(5.0–12)	27.4(20–37)	1.3
48	59.7(39–91)	38.5(20–67)	2.0	20.2(11–32)	42.4(29–60)	1.7
72	96.7(58–166)	75.4(38–142)	2.6	36.8(20–62)	60.6(39–91)	2.0

Δt (h)	D_0	Factor XII D	R	Factor XIII D	D_0	R
0	16.2(12–21)	0.30(0.20–0.40)	1.0	0.05(0.03–0.07)	10.7(9.8–12)	1.0
2	17.1(13–22)	0.62(0.41–0.83)	1.0	0.10(0.07–0.13)	10.8(10–12)	1.0
4	18.0(13–23)	1.27(0.83–1.8)	1.1	0.20(0.14–0.27)	10.9(10–12)	1.0
6	19.0(14–25)	1.96(1.3–2.7)	1.1	0.30(0.21–0.40)	11.0(10–12)	1.0
8	20.0(15–26)	2.69(1.8–3.8)	1.1	0.41(0.28–0.55)	11.1(10–12)	1.0
12	22.0(17–29)	4.25(2.7–6.0)	1.2	0.62(0.40–0.83)	11.3(10–12)	1.0
24	28.6(21–38)	9.77(6.0–14)	1.4	1.27(0.82–1.7)	12.1(11–13)	1.1
48	43.9(31–60)	24.4(13–39)	1.7	2.67(1.7–3.6)	13.4(12–15)	1.1
72	64.4(43–98)	44.8(24–78)	2.1	4.22(2.8–6.0)	15.0(13–17)	1.2

needed for infusions at 48 hour intervals. This fact should be taken into account in cost-benefit calculations of coagulation factor preparations. Highly purified preparations permit frequent injection of small volumes of concentrate and the extra costs involved in purification, or loss in recovered activity, may well be compensated.

A special point concerns the calculation of loading doses in Table 8.12. When it is strictly claimed that plasma levels are not allowed to fall below the target level, a situation occurs as shown in the upper panel of Fig. 8.3. The plasma levels remain

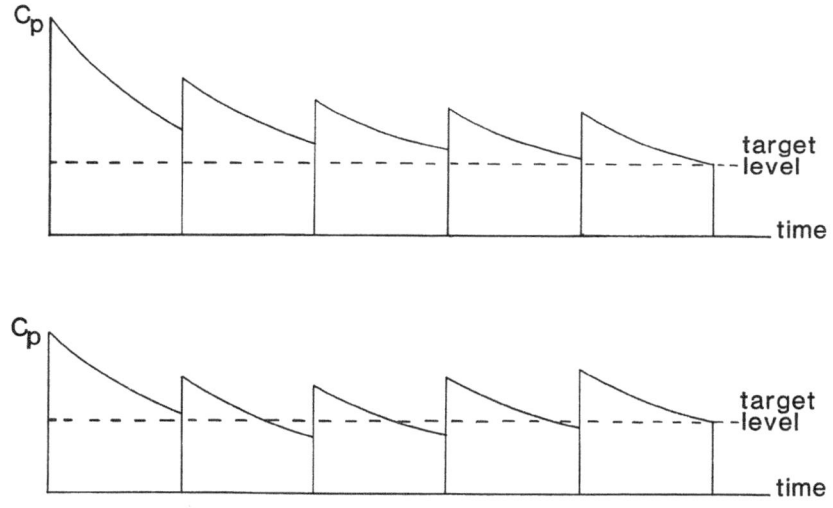

Fig 8.3   Plasma levels during therapy with intermittent doses. Upper panel: levels are not allowed to fall below the target level. Lower panel: levels are allowed to fall slightly below the target level.

above the target level for a considerable period of time and the extra quantity of protein eliminated due to this fact must be provided by the loading dose D_0, resulting in large values of D_0. In the situation shown in the lower panel of Fig. 8.3, plasma levels are allowed to fall slightly below the target level. The reduction of the loading dose in that case is disproportionally

large because the lacking quantity of factor can be compensated
during several cycles. It was calculated that by allowing a 10%
fall below the target level (in the example given this would
imply a temporary drop of plasma levels to 27% of normal) the
loading dose could be reduced by a factor 5 for factor VII and a
factor 1.5 for factor IX. This reduction is most pronounced for
short time intervals. The loading doses D_0 in Table 8.12 were
calculated by allowing such a temporary dip of 10%.

8.5 Complicating factors in dose calculation of coagulation factors

Accurate calculation of dosage schemes in substitution therapy presupposes accurate therapeutic strategies. However, a
recent meeting on the management of the most common disorders in
this field, hemophilia A and B, made it apparent that there is no
common opinion about optimal treatment of joint- and muscle
bleedings which form about 90% of complications in such patients
[242]. This lack of concensus is also apparent from large differences in the quantity of factor VIII needed per patient per year,
even in highly developed countries with home-therapy programs
supervised by treatment centres. Figures quoted for 1975 ranged
from 8750 units and 15000 units for respectively Switzerland and
Norway to 95000 units and 89000 units for Germany and Luxembourg
[242]. In view of these discrepancies it might well be asked if
attempts at accurate dose-calculation are rewarding.

However, clinical practice is more uniform in other situations. It is for instance generally agreed that, during and after
surgery, plasma levels of most coagulation factors should be
maintained at levels between 30% and 50% of normal. Moreover,
figures as quoted for different countries may be misleading
because they refer to in vitro determined activities and it is
well known that in vivo recovery may vary considerably between
different preparations. Low in vivo recovery of factor VIII
concentrates has provoked the statement that purification of
factor VIII leads to increased in vivo elimination rates [242].
Although this may be true for a rapidly eliminated fraction in

the preparation, the remaining fraction of activity after infusion of concentrates has the same fractional catabolic rate
constant as factor VIII from plasma or radiolabeled factor VIII
(cf. Table 8.8). As discussed in Section 8.3, purification could
also not explain the rapid removal of factor VII in approximately
50% of reported cases, because rapid elimination after infusion
of fresh blood and slow elimination after infusion of concentrates were both observed.

Still it is apparent that variable in vivo recovery is a major
obstacle in the realization of accurate dosage schemes. On the
basis of extensive clinical experience, it was emperically found
that injection of one unit of factor VIII per kg of body weight
produces a 2% increase in plasma levels when infused in freshly
frozen plasma and a 1.5% increase in plasma levels when infused
as a factor VIII concentrate [220]. Assuming a mean plasma volume
of 50 ml/kg in these patients, including children, this implies a
100% in vivo recovery for plasma and a 75% in vivo recovery for
concentrate. However 100% recovery of factor VIII concentrates is
also often found. It seems as if in vivo recovery is not only
preparation-dependent but may also be patient-dependent. "Low
responders" are repeatedly described in the literature, also in
the absence of circulating antibodies [242]. Such patient-dependent variations are also suggested by coefficients of variation
as large as 40% for the in vivo recovery of one and the same
batch of concentrate [220]. A figure of 50% is used in the literature for in vivo recovery of factor IX concentrates.

An interesting phenomenon is apparent from data obtained
during prolonged infusion of coagulation factors. The initial
recovery of a factor IX concentrate was approximately 50%, but
from the saturation level in plasma after several days of continuous infusion and the quantity infused, it appears that the in
vivo recovery has increased to approximately 100% [282]. It seems
as if the mechanism responsable for the rapid removal of a fraction of the protein has become saturated after a few days of continuous infusion. A similar observation follows from continuous
infusion of factor VIII [293]. Up to 24 hours an incomplete in
vivo recovery is apparent from the value of FCR = 0.10 h^{-1} as

calculated from the quantity infused and the saturation level reached in plasma. This is clearly an overestimation of the normal value of FCR = 0.065 h^{-1} for factor VIII, indicating the presence of a rapidly eliminated fraction. Estimating the value of FCR by the same procedure after 3-6 days of continuous infusion, however, a value of FCR = 0.066 - 0.079 h^{-1} is obtained and it appears that in vivo recovery has become 100%. Dose-calculation of coagulation factors could also be complicated by increased elimination rates in patients who are actually bleeding due to consumption of coagulation factors in the clotting process. As mentioned in the introduction, there is evidence that this complication does not occur. Turnover studies of radiolabeled factors I, II and VIII in healthy controls have produced similar values for FCR as found from the disappearance from plasma after therapeutic infusion of these factors in bleeding patients (cf. Tables 8.5, 8.6 and 8.8). In patients with hemophilia B it was also shown that FCR was not increased during periods of bleeding [210]. Increased consumption of factor VII during bleeding was suggested in a study reporting a much lower value of FCR in a healthy control infused with factor VII concentrate [209]. However, as discussed in Section 8.3, similar low values of FCR for factor VII are also found in patients.

The high value of FCR used for factor VII in Tables 8.11 and 8.12 implies that therapeutic infusion can only have shortly lasting effects. As shown in Table 8.11, an initial plasma level of 100% factor VII will fall below 1% within approximately 12 hours. Evidence from clinical practice seems to indicate a more prolonged therapeutic effect which might indicate that most factor VII preparations contain fractions of more slowly degraded activity.

Although values of FCR are apparently not increased during bleeding, they may be changed in various clinical situations. Increased values for FCR have been described for factors II, VII, IX and X during fever and hyperthyroidism [281]. Such changes in values of FCR should be added to the biological variation included in Tables 8.11 and 8.12 and this implies that dosage-schemes as calculated from these tables should be considered only as first approximations and should always be checked in practice by repeated determination of coagulation factor levels actually obtained during therapy.

CHAPTER 9

A REVIEW OF DATA ON THE TURNOVER AND DISTRIBUTION

OF CIRCULATING PROTEINS.

Table 9.1 <u>Experimental procedures and observed variables in</u>
<u>studies on circulating proteins</u>.

<u>Procedures</u>:

A Intravenous bolus injection of labeled homologous or autologous
protein preparations in healthy controls.

B Biosynthetic "pulse" labeling with a single intravenous injection or oral dose of labeled protein precursors.

C In vivo labeling by repeated injections, continuous infusions
or prolonged intake of labeled protein precursors.

D Intravenous bulk infusion of homologous proteins in controls or
protein-deficient subjects.

E Measurement of reappearance of proteins in plasma after depletion of the plasma protein pool.

F Study of transient changes in plasma protein concentrations
after various forms of trauma.

G Measurement of the disappearance of proteins from plasma after
blockade of synthesis or removal of the source of production.

<u>Observed variables</u>:

a Protein concentrations in plasma or serum.

b Protein degradation products excreted in urine and faeces.

c Protein concentrations in extravascular fluids such as lymph.

d Externally detectable labels in the body, using for instance
organ scanning or whole-body counting.

e Labeled low-molecular weight substances appearing in plasma or
urine after administration of labeled protein precursors.

Table 9.2 <u>Techniques for the analysis of data obtained in studies</u>
<u>on circulating proteins (cf. Chapter 4 for details)</u>.

1 Exponential analysis of disappearance curves of proteins from
plasma. Unless stated otherwise, double-exponential analysis
was performed.

2 Estimation of catabolic rate constants from urinary excretion
and plasma concentrations of label.

3 Estimation of catabolic rate constants from whole-body counts
and plasma concentrations of label.

4 Estimation of the extravascular protein pool $E(t)$ at "equilibrium time", i.e. when $E(t)$ is maximal.

5 Integration of the plasma disappearance curve after exponential extrapolation in time (Nosslin's method no.1).

6 Integration of the plasma protein curve over short time intervals with separate estimates of the extravascular pool (Nosslin's method no.2).

7 Determination of the diappearance rate of labeled protein from
plasma during the "catabolic phase" after administration of
labeled protein precursors.

8 Estimation of protein synthesis from the production of labeled
protein and the labeled fraction of a low-molecular weight
substance, after injection of labeled precursors.

9 Determination of saturation levels of plasma protein concentrations after continuous intravenous infusion of proteins.

10 Determination of the disappearance rate of protein from plasma during the "catabolic phase" after transient protein release due to trauma.

11 Analysis of transient changes in plasma protein concentrations
together with similar changes of a simultaneously released
protein.

Table 9.3 <u>List of plasma proteins for which ciculatory parameters
have been obtained.</u>

M : relative molecular mass

S : sedimentation constant in water at 20 ^{O}C, expressed in
Svedberg units i.e. 10^{-13} cm/sec/dyne

S_f : flotation constant (-S) in a medium of relative density
1.063 at 26 ^{O}C, expressed in Svedberg units

$S_f(1.21)$: flotation constant in a medium of relative density 1.21
at 26 ^{O}C, expressed in Svedberg units

D : diffusion coefficient in water at 20 ^{O}C, expressed in
10^{-7} cm^2/sec

v_{20} : partial specific volume of the protein dissolved in water at 20 ^{O}C, expressed in ml/g

pI : isoelectric point, i.e. the pH value at which the molecule has no net charge

E_{280} : extinction coefficient, i.e. $\log_{10}(I_0/I)$, for light tra-
velling 1 cm through a solution containing 10 g/l (1%)
of protein, and a wavelength of 280 nm.

CH_2O : carbohydrate content expressed as a percentage of total
mass

<u>I Proteins with transport functions [417,357,529].</u>

protein(abbreviation)	M	S	D	v_{20}	pI	E_{280}	CH_2O
-Prealbumin(PA)	54,980	4.2			4.7	13.2	0
-Albumin(Alb)	66,500	4.6	6.1	0.733	5.8	5.8	0
-Transcortin(TC)	49,500	3.66		0.701		7.1	27
-Thyroxine-binding globulin(TBG)	63,000	3.4			3.8		13
-Retinol-binding protein(RBP)	21,000	2.26					
-Haptoglobin(Hp)							
genetic Hp 1-1	85,000	4.4	4.7	0.766	4.1	12	19.3
variants: Hp 1-2	S = 4.3 - 6.5						
Hp 2-2	S = 7.2 (polymeric)						

	M	S	D	v_{20}	pI	E_{280}	CH_2O
-Ceruloplasmin(Cp)	160,000	7.08	3.76	0.713	4.4	14.9	8
-Hemopexin(Hpx)	57,000	4.8		0.702	5.8	7.0	23
-Transferrin(Tf)	77,000	5.54	5.0	0.758	5.9	19.7	5.9
-Lactoferrin	largely similar to transferrin						

Lipoproteins [324,405,245].

-Very low density lipoprotein(VLDL): density = 0.96-1.006 g/ml

protein content	M	S_f	mass ratio
7-10 %(of mass)	5.10^6-10^7	20-400	apo B/apo C-I/apo C-II/
			apo C-III/apo E = 36.9/
			3.3/6.7/39.9/13 with
			traces of apo A

-Intermediate density lipoprotein(IDL):density = 1.006-1.019 g/ml

protein content	M	S_f	mass ratio
14-18 %	$3.10^6-5.10^6$	12-20	apo B/apo E = 60/30
			contains also apo C

-Low density lipoprotein(LDL): density = 1.019-1.063 g/ml

protein content	M	S_f	mass ratio
22 %	$(2.2-3.5)10^6$	0-12	apo B = 98 % with
			traces of apo C

-High density lipoprotein(LDL): density = 1.063-1.21 g/ml

protein content	M	$S_f(1.21)$	mass ratio
33-59 %	$(148-386)10^3$	0-9	apo A-I/apo A-II/apo
			C-I/apo C-II/apo C-III
			= 67/22/$\pm$2/$\pm$2/$\pm$4

Lipoproteins (continued)	M		CH_2O
-Apoprotein A-I (apo A-I)	28,330		
-Apoprotein A-II (apo A-II)	17,000		
-Apoprotein B (apo B)			5
-Apoprotein C-I (apo C-I)	6,331		
-Apoprotein C-II (apo C-II)	8,837		
-Apoprotein C-III (apo C-III)	8,764		
-Apoprotein D (apo D)	22,100		18
-Apoprotein E (apo E)	33,100		± 10

II Immunoglobulins [520,513,418,453]

	M	S	D	V_{20}	pI	E_{280}	CH_2O
-IgM	900,000	19		0.724		13.3	12
-IgG	150,000	6.6	4.0	0.739		13.8	2.9
-IgA (monomer)	162,000	6.6	3.4	0.725		13.4	7.5
-IgD	172,000	7.0		0.717		14.5	11.3
-IgE	196,000	7.9				14.1	10.7

III Complement factors [10,106,355].

	M	S	D	V_{20}	pI	E_{280}	CH_2O
$-C_{1q}$	400,000	11.1				6.82	8.5
$-C_3$	190,000	9.55		0.736			1.5
$-C_4$	200,000	10.1					6.9
-C5	190,000	8.8					
-Factor B	93,000	6.1	5.4	0.72			
-Beta-1H	150,000	6.4		0.733			

IV Blood coagulation factors [106,226,136].

	M	S	D	V_{20}	pI	E_{280}	CH_2O
-Factor I	341,000	7.63	1.97	0.723	5.5	13.6	2.5
-Factor II	69,000			0.713		± 13.6	8.1
-Factor V	335,000					± 8.9	13
-Factor VII	48,000					± 10	+

	M	S	D	v_{20}	pI	E_{280}	CH_2O
-Factor VIII	$100,000-2.10^6$						+
-Factor IX	57,000			0.713		13.2	17
-Factor X	59,000			0.719		11.6	15
-Factor XI	130,000				8.6	13.4	± 5
-Factor XII	76,000					14.2	16.8

V Enzyme inhibitors [417,104].

	M	S	D	v_{20}	pI	E_{280}	CH_2O
-Alpha$_1$-antitrypsin	50,000	3.5	5.2	0.728	4.0	5.3	12.2

(genetic variants are classified in the (P)roteinase (i)nhibitor system)

	M	S	D	v_{20}	pI	E_{280}	CH_2O
-Alpha$_2$-macroglobulin	750,000	19	2.41	0.728	5.4	8.1	8.4
-Antithrombin III	67,000					6.1	

VI Other proteins [417,103,271].

	M	S	D	v_{20}	pI	E_{280}	CH_2O
-Alpha$_1$-acid glyco-protein	44,000	3.11	5.27	0.675	2.7	8.9	41.4
-Plasminogen	86,000					16.1	
-Alpha-fetoprotein	70,000	4.5	6.2	0.726	4.9	5.3	4

Table 9.4 <u>Circulatory parameters for plasma proteins in man</u>.

C_s : steady-state protein concentration in plasma (g/l)

FCR : fractional catabolic rate constant for the elimination of protein from plasma (h^{-1})

TER : fractional transcapillary escape rate constant (h^{-1})

$(E/P)_s$: steady-state ratio of extra- to intravascular protein pool

k_d : apparent exponential disappearance constant of the final part of the plasma curve (h^{-1}). FCR can be estimated from k_d by using Table 5.1 or Equation 8.2 with $k_2 = k_d$ and average values for TER and $(E/P)_s$

n : number of experiments

Parametervalues are presented as: mean

$\pm$CV(%)

Methods are indicated as: A(a,b,1,2)

A : experimental procedure (cf. Table 9.1)

a,b : observed variables (cf. Table 9.1)

1,2 : methods used for analysis of data (cf Table 9.2)

Values indicated with * were calculated from the original data

-Protein [ref]	method	C_s	FCR	TER	$(E/P)_s$	k_d	n
-Prealbumin							
[338]	A(a,b,1,4)	0.34	0.030		1.0		4
	^{131}I	$\pm$22	$\pm$7		$\pm$10		
[484]	A(a,b,5)	0.31	0.025		1.3		4
	^{131}I;^{125}I	$\pm$9	$\pm$13		$\pm$36		

Table 9.4 (continued)

-Albumin	method	C_s	FCR	TER	$(E/P)_s$	k_d	n
[100] 3-exponential tial curve	A(a,1) [131]I	43.3 ±4	0.0043 ±14	0.013 ±12	0.73 ±15		6
	rapidly equilibrating pool:			0.055 ±29	0.54 ±16		
	A(a,b,2)		0.0034 ±2				4
	A(a,b,4)			$((E_1+E_2)/P)s$:	1.08 ±9		4
[37] 3-exponential tial curve	A(a,1) [131]I	45.1 ±4	0.0052 ±16	0.013* ±28	1.06* ±23	0.0020 ±11	20
	rapidly equilibrating pool:			0.030* ±51	0.34* ±68		
	A(a,b,2)		0.0049 ±17				
	a(a,b,4)			$((E_1+E_2)/P)_s$:	1.17 ±12		
[464] 3-exponen- tial curve	A(a,1) [131]I	41.8 ±4	0.0038 ±11	0.013* ±42	0.93* ±22	0.0015 ±8	13
	rapidly equilibrating pool:			0.020* ±32	0.46* ±39		
[73]	A(a,5) [131]I	47 ±9	0.0048 ±15		1.25 ±6		12
[348] initial phase	A(a,1)	38 ±6	TER_1+TER_2:	0.054 ±20			28
[51]	A(a,b,c,1,2)			0.010	1.33	0.0055	1

These values exclude the intraperitoneal cavity. It was found that catabolism is proportional to plasma albumin levels.

| [159,42] analbumi- nemics | D(a,1) A(a,1) | | | | | 0.0001- 0.0006 | 2 |

Values of FCR decrease for plasma levels below normal

Table 9.4 (continued)

	method	C_s	FCR	TER	$(E/P)_s$	k_d	n
-Thyroxine-binding globulin							
[87] control patients	A(a,b,1,2) ^{125}I	0.022 ±13	0.013[*] ±7		1.25[*] ±19	0.0025 ±24	6
[366] control patients	A(a,b,1,2) $^{125}I;^{131}I$	0.014 ±13	0.014[*] ±7		1.5[*] ±15	0.0024 ±8	9
-Retinol-binding protein							
[484]	A(a,b,5) $^{125}I;^{131}I$	±0.005	±0.80		±4.9		3
-Haptoglobulin							
[161] control patients	A(a,b,1,2) ^{131}I		0.015 ±37				10
[69] control patients	A(a,b,2) $^{131}I;^{125}I$	1.5 ±40	0.0067 ±28				10
[333] hemoglobin infusion	E(a,1)	0.82 ±29	0.013- 0.029				9
[137] ^{14}C-glucosamine ^{35}S-methionine	B(a,10)	0.85 ±33				0.0064 ±24	18
[Chapter 7] patients with AMI	F(a,11)	1.5 ±63	0.011 ±30				11

Comparison of [333](low levels), [161,69](normal levels) and
Chapter 7(high levels) indicates that FCR does not depend on
plasma Hp levels or genetic type of Hp.

Table 9.4 (continued)

	method	C_s	FCR	TER	$(E/P)_s$	k_d	n
-Ceruloplasmin							
[263]	A(a,1)	0.40	0.017		1.5		13
3-exponen-	131I	±15	±24		±16		
tial	control						
	patients						
[452]	D(a,1)					±0.0064	2
aceruloplas-	A(a,1)					±0.0058	
minogenics	67Cu;64Cu						
-Hemopexin							
[419]	E(a,1)					0.0041	1
hematin injections							
[534]	A(a,b,1,2)	0.72	0.0098		2.1	0.0041	10
control	125I	±12	±13		±20	±15	
patients							
[264]	A(a,b,1,2)	0.90	0.012		1.0		9
3-exponen-	125I	±15	±17				
tial	mixed		rapidly equili-				
	patients		brating pool: ±0.5				
-Transferrin							
[247]	A(a,d,1)	2.3	0.0083*	0.019*	0.95*	0.0038	8
	59Fe;131I	±9	±8	±30	±15	±8	
[26]	A(a,b,1,2)	1.9	0.0073*		0.96	0.0033	9
	131I	±24	±27		±9	±10	
[235]	A(a,b,1,2)	2.1	0.0072		1.00		9
	131I	±9	±7		±5		
[254]	B(a,c,8)	2.2	0.0045				7
	14C-carbonate	±8	±42				
-Lactoferrin							
[41]	A(a,5)	0.009	0.24				9
	125I	±38	±17				

Table 9.4 (continued)

Lipoproteins

	method	Cs	FCR	TER	$(E/P)_s$	k_d	n
-VLDL							
[447]	B(a,b,7)	0.067				0.22	5
	75Se-selenomethionine	±48				±20	
[429]	A(a,l)	0.074				0.19	8
	131I-apo B	±48				±44	
[48]	A(a,b,l)	0.055	0.18				4
	125I-apo B	±36	±34				
-LDL							
[273]	A(a,b,1,5)	0.62	0.019		0.46		10
	125I-LDL	±35	±16		±6		
	A(a,b,2)		0.018				
			±21				
[344]	A(a,b,1,2)	0.98	0.013		0.25		5
	125I-apo B	±17	±9		±3		
[84]	A(a,l)	0.73	0.012		0.67		5
	131I-LDL	±19	±12		±16		
	A(a,b,6)		0.013		0.56		
			±6		±28		
	A(a,d,6)		0.013		0.61		
			±5		±10		
	A(a,b,2)		0.012				
			±28				
	A(a,b,4)				0.47		
					±7		
	A(a,d,4)				0.49		
					±10		
-HDL							
[64]	A(a,b,l)	0.36	0.0047	0.013	0.62		8
	125I-apo A	±22	±24	±21	±19		

Elimination occurs partly extravascular: k_e=0.0061±23 h^{-1} (cf. Chapter 4)

Table 9.4 (continued)

Immunoglobulins

	method	C_s	FCR	TER	$(E/P)_s$	k_d	n
-IgM [336] mixed patients	A(a,b,1,2) ^{131}I		0.0032 ±14	0.0055 ±23	0.35 ±32		7
[236] control patients	A(a,b,1,2) ^{131}I	0.58 ±28	0.0044 ±14		0.36 ±15		28

FCR does not depend on plasma IgM concentrations, as also found in ref.[32].

	method	C_s	FCR	TER	$(E/P)_s$	k_d	n
[533] control patients	A(a,b,1,2) $^{131}I;^{125}I$	1.3 ±55	0.0063 ±19		0.71 ±10		12
-IgG [99]	A(a,1) $^{131}I;^{125}I$	11.0 ±8	0.0028 ±25	0.011 ±19	0.85 ±23	0.0013 ±15	10
	A(a,b,2)		0.0025 ±28				
	A(a,b,4)				1.0 ±15		
[8]	A(a,b,6) $^{131}I;^{125}I$		0.0025* ±40	0.010 ±47	0.93* ±41		12

Data indicate partial extravascular elimination with a true value of FCR=0.0016 h^{-1} and k_e=0.0011 h^{-1} (cf. Chapter 4)

	method	C_s	FCR	TER	$(E/P)_s$	k_d	n
[15] control patients	A(a,b,5) ^{131}I	13 ±13	0.0026 ±22	0.016 ±30	0.92 ±13	0.0016 ±18	21
[162]	A(a,b,2,4) ^{131}I	11.0 ±9	0.0023 ±7	0.011 ±11	0.98 ±11		12
-IgG$_1$ [309] myeloma proteins	A(a,b,1,2) $^{11}I;^{125}I$	6.9 ±30	0.0033 ±25		0.96 ±8	0.0014 ±25	6

Table 9.4 (continued)

	method	C_s	FCR	TER	(E/P)s	k_d	n
-IgG$_2$			0.0029		0.89	0.0014	4
			±4		±11	±9	
-IgG$_3$		0.5	0.0070		0.56	0.0041	6
		±34	±4		±9	±10	
-IgG$_4$			0.0028		0.85	0.0014	5
			±15		±9	±13	

FCR decreases for low plasma IgG levels and may increase to twice its normal value for elevated levels (cf. also [162])

	method	C_s	FCR	TER	(E/P)s	k_d	n
-IgA [456] control patients	A(a,b,1,2) ^{131}I;^{125}I	2.5 ±55	0.011 ±15		1.4 ±35		12
[310]	A(a,b,1,2) ^{131}I;^{125}I	2.3 ±22	0.010 ±10		0.83 ±7	0.0049 ±8	7
-IgA$_2$		0.32 ±25	0.013 ±13		0.75 ±4	0.0064 ±7	7
-IgD [387] control patients	A(a,1) ^{125}I	0.04 ±85	0.016 ±27		0.36 ±8	0.010 ±36	12
-IgE [224,514]	A(a,b,5)	17.10$^-$ ±86	0.039 ±27		1.46 ±29	0.011 ±29	10

Data indicate partial extravascular elimination with true FCR= 0.027^*h^{-1} and $k_e = 0.008^*h^{-1}$

Table 9.4 (continued)

	method	C_s	FCR	TER	$(E/P)_s$	k_d	n
Complement factors							
$-C_{1q}$							
[261]	A(a,b,1,2) ^{125}I	±0.17	±0.28		±0.6		2
$-C_3$							
[352]	A(a,b,5) ^{125}I	1.34 ±13	0.021 ±13		0.65 ±25	0.013 ±20	13
[91]	A(a,1) ^{125}I	1.17 ±14	0.016 ±8		0.35 ±40		11
	A(a,b,2)		0.016 ±11				
	A(a,b,6)		0.017 ±11				
[398]	A(a,b,1,2) $^{125}I; ^{131}I$	1.4 ±19	0.017 ±10				20
$-C4$							
[86]	A(a,b,1,2) $^{125}I; ^{131}I$	0.58 ±21	0.018 ±25		0.52 ±63		11
[398]	A(a,b,1,2) $^{125}I; ^{131}I$	0.48 ±33	0.014 ±8				9
$-C5$							
[398]	A(a,b,1,2) $^{125}I; ^{131}I$	±0.1	±0.019				3
[430]	A(a,b,6) ^{125}I	0.11 ±12	0.018 ±12		0.49 ±39		7
	A(a,1)		0.017 ±10		0.44 ±34		7
	A(a,b,2)		0.017 ±9				7
$-$Factor B							
[90]	A(a,b,1,2) ^{125}I	0.3 ±35	0.017 ±10		0.35 ±29		11

Table 9.4 (continued)

	method	C_s	FCR	TER	$(E/P)_s$	k_d	n
-Beta-1H							
[92]	A(a,b,6)	0.71	0.013		0.52	0.0091	7
	^{125}I	±11	±14		±19	±9	

Data indicate partial extravascular elimination

Blood coagulation factors

	method	C_s	FCR	TER	$(E/P)_s$	k_d	n
-Factor I (fibrinogen)							
[Chapter 8]	various	2.0-	0.010	0.025	0.20		several
	methods	3.6	±10	±40	±25		studies
-Factor II (prothrombin)							
[Chapter 8]	various	0.06-	0.018	0.030	0.55		several
	methods	0.17	±20	±50	±25		studies
-Factor V							
[Chapter 8]	,,	0.007-	±0.07	±0.025	±0.20		,,
		0.013					
-Factor VII							
[Chapter 8]	,,	0.0005-	±0.40	±0.050	±0.80		,,
		0.0006					
-Factor VIII							
[Chapter 8]	,,		0.065	0.025	0.20		,,
			±30				
-Factor IX							
[Chapter 8]	,,	0.004-	0.050	0.050	0.80		,,
		0.005	±30	±50	±35		
-Factor X							
[Chapter 8]	,,	0.007-	±0.04	±0.05	±0.8		,,
		0.008					
-Factor XI							
[Chapter 8]	,,	0.002-	±0.02	±0.02	±0.8		,,
		0.004					
-Factor XII							
[Chapter 8]	,,		±0.005	±0.025	±0.2		,,

Table 9.4 (continued)

Data for factors I, II, VIII, and IX, indicate that FCR is not dependent on plasma concentrations of these factors

Enzyme inhibitors

	method	C_s	FCR	TER	$(E/P)_s$	k_d	n
-alpha$_1$-antitrypsin							
[296]	D(a,1)	2.3-				0.0051	3
P$_1$-- and P$_i$ZZ subjects		4.2				+10	
[275]	A(a,b,5)		0.012		1.39	0.0042	4
	125$_I$;131$_I$		+10		+13	+8	
[241]	A(a,b,6)	2.3	0.014	0.033	1.1	0.0063	7
	125$_I$;131$_I$	+36	+11	+32	+17	+12	

Comparison of refs[296,275,241] indicates that values of FCR do not depend on genetic type

[Chapter 7]	F(a,11)	2.4	0.015				11
patients with AMI		+14	+88				

Comparison of [296],low levels, [275,241],normal levels, and Chapter 7, high levels, indicates that FCR does not depend on plasma alpha$_1$-antitrypsin levels

	method	C_s	FCR	TER	$(E/P)_s$	k_d	n
-Alpha$_2$-macroglobulin							
[375]	A(a,1)		0.0044	0.012	0.46	0.0028	6
	131$_I$		+14	+14	+20	+15	
[259]	A(a,1)	2.8				0.0030	7
	131$_I$	+20				+18	
[147]	A(a,b,2,4)	2.1	0.0064		0.60	0.0034	4
	131$_I$	+15	+20		+25	+15	
-Antithrombin III							
[104]	A(a,b,1,2)	0.20	0.023	0.021	0.84*	0.010	4
	125$_I$	+12	+4	+20	+13	+9	

Table 9.4 (continued)

Other proteins

	methods	C_s	FCR	TER	$(E/P)_s$	k_d	n
-Alpha$_1$-acid glycoprotein							
[519]	A(a,b,2)	1.1	0.0066			0.0052	7
	^{131}I	± 34	± 10			± 14	
[540]	B(a,b,10)	± 0.8				0.0083	4
patients	^{14}C-glucosamine						
after							
burns							
[Chapter 7]	F(a,11)	0.64	0.0087				11
patients with AMI		± 20	± 50				
-Plasminogen							
[103]	A(a,b,1,2)	0.21	0.023	0.012	0.40*	0.013	12
	^{125}I;^{131}I	± 9	± 16	± 38	± 26	± 13	
-Alpha-fetoprotein							
[271]	G(a,1)	8.10^{-6}				0.005	vari-
post partum		± 50				± 25	ous
							studies

Table 9.5 <u>Circulatory parameters for plasma proteins in the dog, rabbit and rat.</u>

Symbols are explained in Table 9.4

-Prealbumin	method	C_s	FCR	TER	$(E/P)_s$	k_d	n
rat[350]	A(a,1) 125I	0.34 ±6				0.065 ±15	
-Albumin							
dog[523]	A(a,1) 131I	33.4 ±7	0.0074 ±5	0.034 ±23	1.09 ±18	0.0033 ±10	6
rabbit[98]	A(a,b,1,2) 131I		0.0083 ±16		1.44 ±11	0.0034 ±9	5
rat[27]	A(a,b,2) 131I		0.029 ±14		1.02 ±25		16
rat[378]	A(a,1) 125I			0.13* ±14			11
-Transcortin							
rat[215]	A(a,1) 125I					±0.17	4
-Retinol-binding protein							
rat[350]	A(a,1) 125I	0.065 ±14				0.11 ±15	5
-Ceruloplasmin							
rabbit[109]	A(a,1) 125I					±0.012	2
rat[350]	A(a,1) 125I	0.33 ±6				0.028 ±8	5
-Hemopexin							
rabbit[272]	A(a,1) 125I	0.44 ±35	0.067 ±15	0.092 ±30	0.80 ±25	0.031 ±23	18
rabbit[109]	A(a,1) 125I		±0.08	±0.07*	±0.9	±0.03	2
rat[272]	A(a,1) 125I					±0.013	3

Table 9.5 (continued)

-Transferrin	method	C_s	FCR	TER	$(E/P)_s$	k_d	n
rabbit[426]	A(a,1) 125I		0.018		1.27	0.0069	6
			±13		±7	±14	
rat[173]	A(a,b,1) 131I		±0.023		±1.5	±0.007	8
-High density lipoprotein							
dog[314]	A(a,1) 125I					0.0083	4
						±20	
rat[388]	A(a,1) 125I					±0.066	4
-Immunoglobulin M							
rabbit[402]	A(a,1) 125I	0.57	0.017		0.41	0.0096	10
		±22	±16		±18	±11	
rat[349]	A(a,1) 125I					0.028	8
						±14	
-Immunoglobulin G							
dog[14]	A(a,1) 125I	9.9	0.0085	0.018	0.72	0.0041	10
		±12	±23	±25	±31	±23	
rabbit[402]	A(a,1) 125I	9.7	0.010		0.96	0.0048	12
		±21	±14		±14	±12	
rat[349]	A(a,1) 125I					IgG_1: ±0.013	4
						IgG_2: ±0.0065	3
-Immunoglobulin A							
rat[349]	A(a,1) 125I					0.026	5
						±16	
-Factor I (fibrinogen)							
dog[279]	A(a,1) 131I					0.012	20
						±13	
rabbit[368]	A(a,d,1) 131I;125I	2.8	0.016	0.019	0.24	0.012	10
		±20	±15	±40	±33	±10	

FCR and TER are not dependent on plasma Fg levels

rabbit[93]	A(a,b,1,2) 131I;125I	2.7	0.019	0.033	0.23		13
		±13	±12	±95	±46		

FCR decreases slightly with increasing body weight

Table 9.5 (continued)

	method	C_s	FCR	TER	$(E/P)_s$	k_d	n
rat[322]	A(a,1)	2.5	0.039	0.056	0.25*	0.030	5
	125I	±12	±33	±25	±20	±7	

-Factor II(prothrombin)

	method	C_s	FCR	TER	$(E/P)_s$	k_d	n
dog[343]	A(a,b,1,2)					0.020*	9
	125I					±20	
dog[199]	G(a,1)					0.017	16
vit.K antagonist						±19	
rat[498]	G(a,1)					0.12	16
vit.K antagonist						±15	

-Factor VII

	method	C_s	FCR	TER	$(E/P)_s$	k_d	n
dog[138]	D(a,1)					0.55	4
	plasma					±30	
	D(a,1)					0.25	18
	blood					±37	
dog[199]	G(a,1)					0.11	16
vit.K antagonist						±19	

The rate of disappearance is probably underestimated (cf.Chapter 8)

-Alpha$_1$-antitrypsin

	method	C_s	FCR	TER	$(E/P)_s$	k_d	n
rabbit[369]	A(a,1)					"F-type":0.010	9
	131I;125I					±11	
						"S-type":0.013	
						±15	

-Alpha$_2$-macroglobulin

	method	C_s	FCR	TER	$(E/P)_s$	k_d	n
rabbit[502]	A(a,1)					"type 1":±0.006	
	131I					"type 2":±0.010	

-Antithrombin III

	method	C_s	FCR	TER	$(E/P)_s$	k_d	n
dog[260]	A(a,b,1,2)	0.58	0.025	0.042	0.69	0.014	20
	125I	±19	±7	±20	±9	±4	

-Alpha-fetoprotein

	method	C_s	FCR	TER	$(E/P)_s$	k_d	n
rat[422]	A(a,d,1)	3.10^{-5}				±0.029	5
	125I	±50					

Table 9.6 <u>List of tissue enzymes mentioned in the text or in</u>
<u>Tables 9.7 and 9.8</u>.

EC : Enzyme Commission code
M : relative molecular mass
localization : if not mentioned, the enzyme is widely distributed
or intracellular localization is uncertain [M.
Dixon, E.C.Webb: Enzymes. London, 1979, 3rd ed]

A <u>Carbohydrate metabolis</u>m

1 Glycolysis	M	localization
-Hexokinase(HK) EC 2.7.1.1	100,000	
-Phosphorylase b EC 2.4.1.1	185,000- 370,000	cytoplasm
-Phosphoglucomutase(PGM) EC 2.7.5.1	62,000	cytoplasm
-Glucosephosphate isomerase(GPI) EC 5.3.1.9	134,000	
-Aldolase(ALD) EC 4.1.2.13	160,000	skeletal muscle cytoplasm
-Glycerol-3-phosphate dehydrogenase (GPDH) EC 1.1.1.8	63,000	
-Glyceraldehyde-phosphate dehydro- genase(GAPDH) EC 1.2.1.12	144,000	cytoplasm
-Pyruvate kinase(PK) EC 2.7.1.40	230,000	
-Lactate dehydrogenase(LDH) EC 1.1.1.27	136,000	cytoplasm
-Alpha-hydroxybutyrate dehydro- genase(HBDH) EC 1.1.1.27	136,000	erythrocytes, heart, kidney

2 Citric acid cycle	M	localization
-Citrate synthase EC 4.1.3.7	100,000	
-NAD$^+$-isocitrate dehydrogenase (ICDH-NAD) EC 1.1.1.41		liver,heart mitochondria
-NADP$^+$-isocitrate dehydrogenase (ICDH-NADP) EC1.1.1.42	60,000	cytoplasm and mitochondria
-Succinate dehydrogenase EC 1.3.99.1		mitochondria
-Malate dehydrogenase(MDH) EC 1.1.1.37	70,000	cytoplasm and mitochondria

3 Hexose monophosphate pathway		
-Phosphogluconate dehydrogenase (PGDH) EC 1.1.1.43	102,000- 129,000	
-Glucose-6-phosphate dehydrogenase (G6PDH) EC 1.1.1.49	210,000	cytoplasm

4 Other enzymes		
-Alpha-amylase EC 3.2.1.1	50,000	pancreas
-Lysozyme EC 3.2.1.17	14,000	
-Beta-N-acetyl glucosaminidase (NAG) EC 3.2.1.30	280,000	lysosomes
-Beta-glucoronidase EC 3.2.1.31	218,000	lysosomes

B Esterases		
-Lipase EC 3.1.1.3		pancreas
-Alkaline phosphatase(AP) EC 3.1.3.1	190,000	cell membrane

	M	localization
-Acid phophatase EC 3.1.3.2	96,000	prostate, erythrocytes lysosomes

C <u>Amino acid metabolism</u>

	M	localization
-Alanine aminotransferase(ALT) EC 3.6.1.2	115,000	liver
-L-leucyl-beta-naphtylamidase (LBNA) EC 3.4.11.1	255,000- 327,000	cell membrane
-Aspartate aminotransferase(AST) EC 2.6.1.1	100,000	cytoplasm and mitochondria
-Cathepsin D EC 3.4.23.5	56,000	lysosomes
-Glutamate dehydrogenase(GLDH) EC 1.4.1.3	2,000,000	liver, mitochondria
-Gamma-glutamyl transpeptidase (gamma-GT) EC 2.3.2.2		cell membrane
-Ornithine carbamyl transferase (OCT) EC 2.1.3.3	108,000	liver

D <u>Other enzymes</u>

	M	localization
-Adenylate kinase(myokinase) (MK) EC 2.7.4.3	21,000	muscle
-Creatine kinase(CK) EC 2.7.3.2	80,000	muscle (CK-MM) heart (CK-MB) brain (CK-BB)
-Cytochrome oxydase EC 1.9.3.1		mitochondria

E <u>Non-enzymatic tissue proteins</u>

	M	localization
-Myoglobin	17,000	muscle, cytoplasm

Table 9.7 <u>Circulatory parameters for tissue enzymes in man.</u>

C_s : normal steady-state activity in plasma (U/l). Values of
C_s vary considerably with assay conditions.

Other symbols are explained in Table 9.4

-Enzyme [ref.]	method	C_s	FCR	TER	$(E/P)_s$	k_d	n
-Phosphoglucomutase							
[120]	D(a,l)	50				0.18	1
-Glucosephosphate isomerase							
[528;Ch.6]	F(a,11)	28	0.27				14
		±28	±37				
-Aldolase							
[120]	D(a,l)	12				0.008	1
-Pyruvate kinase							
[120]	D(a,l)	19				0.046	1
-Lactate dehydrogenase							
[120]	D(a,l)	175			slow phase:	0.017	1
					rapid phase:	0.10	

Slow phase is probably LDH_1/LDH_2 and rapid phase LDH_5

-Alpha-hydroxybutyrate dehydrogenase							
[527]	F(a,11)	80	0.015	0.017	0.80		30
		±19	±44	±64	±62		
-Malate dehydrogenase							
[120]	D(a,l)	50				0.058	1
-Lysozyme							
[186]	A(a,5)	0.009	0.76				9
	^{125}I	±16 g/l	±12				
-Alkaline phosphatase							
[95]	D(a,l)	7**	0.0074	0.028	0.70	0.0047	7
		±56	±25	±35	±30	±23	

**:King-Armstrong units

Table 9.7 (continued)

	method	C_s	FCR	TER	$(E/P)_s$	k_d	n
-Alanine aminotransferase							
[Chapter 6]	F(a,11)	7.0 ± 25	0.042 ± 45				14
-Aspartate aminotransferase (cytoplasmic)							
[120]	D(a,1)	20				0.16	1
[528,Ch.6]	F(a,11)	8.8 ± 26	0.093 ± 26				14
-Adenylate kinase							
[403]	D(a,1)				slow phase:± 0.26 rapid phase:± 2.6		2
-Creatine kinase (CK-MM)							
[120]	D(a,1)	5				0.15	1
[479]	D(a,1)					0.12	6
[527,CH.6]	F(a,11)	37 ± 43	0.20 ± 60				30
-Creatine kinase (CK-MB)							
[528,Ch.6]	F(a,11)		0.34 ± 91				16
-Myoglobin							
[458]	A(a,b,1) 125_I	14.10^{-6} ± 50 g/l	± 0.73*			± 0.037	6

Remark: values of k_d for the enzymes in this table are considerably higher than often quoted in the literature [12,29]. These quoted values were calculated from method F(a,10) and have probably contained error due to continuing release of enzymes (cf. Section 4.4).

Table 9.8 <u>Circulatory parameters for tissue enzymes in the dog,</u>
<u>rabbit and rat.</u>

Symbols are explained in Tables 9.7 and 9.4.

	method	C_s	FCR	TER	$(E/P)_s$	k_d	n
-Glucosephosphate isomerase							
dog[528]	D(a,1)	66	0.36				12
		±33	±33				
-Aldolase							
rat[165]	D(a,1)					0.16	7
						±25	
rabbit[407]	A(a,1)					0.21	4
-Pyruvate kinase							
rat[165]	D(a,1)					0.12	8
						±31	
-Lactate dehydrogenase(LDH_1)							
dog[30]	D(a,1)					0.21	4
						±48	
-Lactate dehydrogenase(LDH_5)							
dog[30]	D(a,1)					0.86	3
rabbit[358]	D(a,5)		0.30			0.20	5
			±33			±14	
rat[165]	D(a,1)					0.77	5
						±10	
-Malate dehydrogenase							
dog[30]	D(a,1)					0.27	5
						±34	

Approx. equal values of k_d for mitochondrial and cytoplasmic MDH

rabbit[11]	D(a,1)					0.27	6
						±27	
rat[165]	D(a,1)					1.20	6
						±21	

Table 9.8 (continued)

	method	C_s	FCR	TER	$(E/P)_s$	k_d	n
-Alpha-amylase							
dog[18]	D(a,1)					0.22 ±31	13
-Lysozyme							
rat[185]	A(a,5) ^{131}I	0.012 ±21	3.6 ±32			0.55 ±35	9
-Lipase							
dog[18]	D(a,1)					0.24 ±34	13
-Alkaline phosphatase							
dog[163]	D(a,1)					±0.014	8
-Alanine aminotransferase							
dog[154]	D(a,1)	14 (37 °C)	0.021* ±12	0.008* ±74	0.33* ±50	0.011 ±16	6
dog[528]	D(a,1)	13 ±49	0.022 ±22	0.031 ±40	0.48 ±30	0.013 ±18	6
rabbit[11]	D(a,1)					0.14 ±28	7
rat[165]	D(a,1)					0.16 ±20	8
-Aspartate aminotransferase(cytoplasmic)							
dog[506]	D(a,10)		0.21 ±19			0.20 ±19	8
dog[511]	D(a,1)					0.18 ±15	8
rabbit[11]	D(a,1)					0.27 ±17	7
rat[165]	D(a,1)					0.30 ±28	8
-Aspartate aminotransferase(mitochondrial)							
dog[155]	D(a,1)					0.85 ±14	8

Table 9.8 (continued)

	method	C_s	FCR	TER	$(E/P)_s$	k_d	n
-Glutamate dehydrogenase							
rat[165]	D(a,l)					0.17	9
						± 21	
-Ornithine carbamyl transferase							
dog[370]	D(a,l)	48				± 0.09	5
		± 42					
-Adenylate kinase							
rat[165]	D(a,l)					0.82	7
						± 62	
-Creatine kinase(CK-MM)							
dog[359]	D(a,l)					0.39	6
						± 28	
dog[382]	D(a,l)					0.29	30
						± 20	
dog[506]	D(a, 9)	60	0.36			0.37	10
		± 44	± 25			± 21	
		$(37\ ^{\circ}C)$					
rat[165]	D(a,l)					1.3	8
						± 20	
-Creatine kinase(CK-MB)							
dog[359]	D(a,l)					0.51	6
						± 26	
-Creatine kinase(CK-BB)							
dog[359]	D(a,l)					0.96	6
						± 37	

APPENDIX

Laplace transforms

For a function $f(t)$, defined for $t \geq 0$, with the property

$$\int_0^\infty e^{-st} |f(t)| \, dt < \infty \quad \text{for } s \geq s_0$$

the Laplace transform $\bar{f}(s)$ is defined by

$$\bar{f}(s) = \int_0^\infty e^{-st} f(t) \, dt \quad (s \geq s_0) \tag{A1}$$

The following properties of the Laplace transformation are extensively used:

$$\bar{f}_1(s) = \bar{f}_2(s), \; s \geq s_0 \qquad \rightarrow f_1(t) = f_2(t) \tag{A2}$$

$$g(t) = \int_0^t f(\tau) \, d\tau \qquad \rightarrow \bar{g}(s) = \bar{f}(s)/s \tag{A3}$$

$$g(t) = \frac{d}{dt} f(t) \qquad \rightarrow \bar{g}(s) = s \, \bar{f}(s) - f(o) \tag{A4}$$

$$f(t) = e^{-kt} \qquad \rightarrow \bar{g}(s) = 1/(s+k) \tag{A5}$$

$$g(t) = \int_0^t f_1(\tau) f_2(t-\tau) \, d\tau \rightarrow \bar{g}(s) = \bar{f}_1(s) \cdot \bar{f}_2(s) \tag{A6}$$

$$f(t) = \delta(t-t_0); \; t_0 \geq o \qquad \rightarrow \bar{f}(s) = e^{-st_0} \tag{A7}$$

Roots of quadratic and cubic equations

The quadratic equation: $x^2 + a_1 x + a_0 = o$

has the roots $x_{1,2} = \frac{1}{2}(-a_1 \pm \sqrt{a_1^2 - 4a_0})$ \hfill (A8)

If $a_1^2 - 4a_0 > 0$ both roots are real

$a_1^2 - 4a_0 = 0$ both roots coincide

$a_1^2 - 4a_0 < 0$ both roots are complex conjugate.

The cubic equation: $x^3 + a_2x^2 + a_1x + a_0 = 0$

has the roots $x_1 = s_1 + s_2 - a_2/3$

$$x_{2,3} = -(s_1+s_2)/2 - a_2/3 \pm i\sqrt{3}(s_1-s_2)/2 \qquad \text{(A9)}$$

with $s_1 = (r + \sqrt{q^3+r^2})^{1/3}$; $s_2 = (r - \sqrt{q^3+r^2})^{1/3}$

$q = a_1/3 - a_2^2/9$; $r = a_1a_2/6 - a_0/2 - a_2^3/27$

If $q^3 + r^2 > 0$ one root is real; two roots are complex conjugate

$q^3 + r^2 = 0$ all roots are real and at least two roots coincide

$q^3 + r^2 < 0$ all roots are real.

<u>The two-compartment model</u>

The changes in time of the
plasma pool $P(t)$ and the
extra-vascular pool $E(t)$
in the model presented
in Fig. A1 are given by:

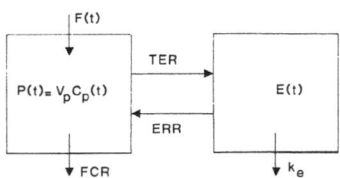

Fig. A.1. General two-compartment
model with intravascular
input.

$$\frac{d}{dt} P(t) = -(FCR+TER)\ P(t) + ERR.E(t) + F(t)$$

$$\frac{d}{dt} E(t) = -(k_e+ERR)\ E(t) + TER.p(t) \qquad \text{(A10)}$$

Laplace-tranformation of these equations gives:

$$(s + FCR + TER)\ \overline{P}(s) - ERR.\overline{E}(s) = \overline{F}(s)$$

$$(s + k_e + ERR)\ \overline{E}(s) = TER.\overline{P}(s)$$

For a bolus injection of one unit of protein at t=0 we have (cf.
(A7)) $\overline{F}(s) = 1$ and one obtains:

$$\bar{P}_b(s) = \frac{s + k_e + ERR}{(s+FCR+TER)(s+k_e+ERR) - TER.ERR} = \frac{P_1}{s+k_1} + \frac{P_2}{s+k_2}$$

$$(A11)$$

$$\bar{E}_b(s) = \frac{TER}{(s+FCR+TER)(s+k_e+ERR) - TER.ERR} = \frac{R_1}{s+k_1} + \frac{R_2}{s+k_2}$$

with $k_{1,2} = \frac{1}{2}(H_1 \pm \sqrt{H_1^2 - 4H_2})$

$H_1 = FCR + TER + ERR + k_e$

$H_2 = FCR . ERR + FCR.k_e + TER.k_e$

In order to express P_1 and P_2 in the model parameters, equation (A11) is written as

$$\frac{s + k_e + ERR}{(s+FCR+TER)(s+k_e+ERR) - TER.ERR} = \frac{P_1(s+k_2) + P_2(s+k_1)}{(s + k_1)(s + k_2)}$$

$$(A13)$$

$$\frac{TER}{(s+FCR+TER)(s+k_e+ERR) - TER.ERR} = \frac{R_1(s+k_2) + R_2(s+k_1)}{(s + k_1)(s + k_2)}$$

The numerators of equations (A13) must be equal, also for special values of s. For $s=-k_1$ and $s=-k_2$ one obtains respectively:

$-k_1 + k_e + ERR = P_1(k_2-k_1)$; $TER = R_1(k_2-k_1)$

$-k_2 + k_e + ERR = P_2(k_1-k_2)$; $TER = R_2(k_1-k_2)$

These expressions can be written as:

$P_1 = (ERR + k_e - k_1)/(k_2 - k_1)$; $P_2 = 1 - P_1$

$$(A14)$$

$R_1 = TER/(k_2-k_1)$; $R_2 = -R_1$

From equation (A11) and the property (A5) it follows that the response curves to a bolus injection of one unit of protein can be written as:

$$P_b(t) = P_1 e^{-k_1 t} + P_2 e^{-k_2 t} ; \quad E_b(t) = R_1 e^{-k_1 t} + R_2 e^{-k_2 t}$$

$$(A15)$$

where P_1, P_2, k_1 and k_2 can be calculated from the model parameters by use of equations (A12) and (A14).

We now consider the reverse problem, i.e. calculation of the model parameters from the response curve observed after a bolus injection of protein. From the equality of the numerators in equations (A13) it can be immediately concluded that:

$$\text{TER} = R_1(k_2-k_1) \; ; \; \text{ERR} + k_e = P_1k_2 + P_2k_1 \tag{A16}$$

The denumerators in equations (A13) also must be equal for special values of s. Chosing the value $s = -(k_e+\text{ERR}) = -(P_1k_2 + P_2k_1)$ one obtains:

$$\text{TER.ERR} = -(P_1k_2 + P_2k_1 - k_1)(P_1k_2 + P_2k_1 - k_2)$$

$$= -P_1(k_2-k_1) \cdot P_2(-k_2+k_1) = P_1P_2(k_2-k_1)^2 \tag{A17}$$

$$\overset{\uparrow}{P_1} = 1-P_2$$

Chosing the value s=0 one obtains:

$$(\text{FCR+TER})(k_e+\text{ERR}) - \text{TER.ERR} = k_1k_2$$

or $\quad \text{FCR}(k_e+\text{ERR}) + k_e.\text{TER} = k_1k_2 \tag{A18}$

Using equations (A16), (A17) and (A18), the model parameters TER, ERR, k_e and FCR can be calculated from the parameters P_1, P_2, k_1 and k_2 obtained from the plasma disappearance curve.

The three-compartment model

The changes in time of the plasma pool P(t) and the extravascular pools $E_1(t)$ and $E_2(t)$ of the model presented in Fig. A2, are given by:

$$\frac{d}{dt}P(t) = -(\text{FCR+TER}_1+\text{TER}_2)P(t) + \text{ERR}_1.E_1(t) + \text{ERR}_2.E_2(t)$$

$$\frac{d}{dt}E_1(t) = -(k_{e1}+k_{12}+\text{ERR}_1)E_1(t) + k_{21}.E_2(t) + \text{TER}_1.P(t) \tag{A19}$$

$$\frac{d}{dt}E_2(t) = -(k_{e2}+k_{21}+\text{ERR}_2)E_2(t) + k_{12}.E_1(t) + \text{TER}_2.P(t)$$

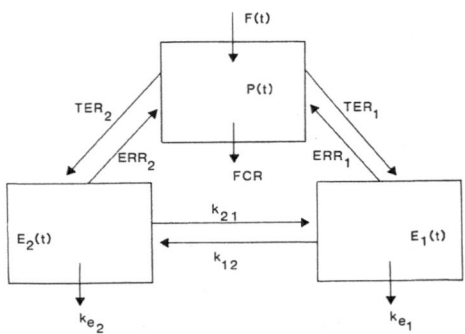

Fig. A.2. General three-compartment model with intravascular input.

Laplace transformation of these equations gives:

$$(s+K_o)\overline{P}(s) = ERR_1 . \overline{E}_1(s) + ERR_2 . \overline{E}_2(s) + \overline{F}(s) \quad ; \quad K_o = FCR + TER_1 + TER_2$$

$$(s+K_1)\overline{E}_1(s) = k_{21} . \overline{E}_2(s) + TER_1 . \overline{P}(s) \quad ; \quad K_1 = k_{e1} + k_{12} + ERR_1$$

$$(s+K_2)\overline{E}_2(s) = k_{12} . \overline{E}_1(s) + TER_2 . \overline{P}(s) \quad ; \quad K_2 = k_{e2} + k_{21} + ERR_2$$

$$(A20)$$

Solving the last two equations for $\overline{E}_1(s)$ and $\overline{E}_2(s)$ and substituting these solutions in the first equation, one obtains:

$$\overline{P}(s) = \frac{(s+a_1)(s+a_2)\ \overline{F}(s)}{(s+K_o)(s+a_1)(s+a_2) - ERR_1(A_1 s+B_1) - ERR_2(A_2 s+B_2)}$$

$$\overline{E}_1(s) = \frac{A_1 s + B_1}{(s+a_1)(s+a_2)}\ \overline{P}(s) \qquad\qquad (A21)$$

$$\overline{E}_2(s) = \frac{A_2 s + B_2}{(s+a_1)(s+a_2)}\ \overline{P}(s)$$

with $a_{1,2} = \tfrac{1}{2}(H_1 \pm \sqrt{H_1^2 - 4H_2})$; $H_1 = K_1 + K_2$; $H_2 = K_1 . K_2 - k_{12} . k_{21}$

$A_1 = TER_1$; $B_1 = TER_1 . K_2 + k_{21} . TER_2$

$$A_2 = TER_2 \; ; \; B_2 = TER_2 \cdot K_1 + k_{12} \cdot TER_1$$

Let $-k_1$, $-k_2$ and $-k_3$ be the roots of the equation:

$$(s+K_o)(s+a_1)(s+a_2) - ERR_1 \cdot (A_1 s+B_1) - ERR_2 \cdot (A_2 s+B_2) =$$

$$= s^3 + H_2 s^2 + H_1 s + H_o = 0 \tag{A22}$$

with $H_o = K_o a_1 a_2 - ERR_1 \cdot B_1 - ERR_2 \cdot B_2$

$\quad\quad H_1 = K_o a_1 + K_o a_2 + a_1 a_2 - ERR_1 \cdot A_1 - ERR_2 \cdot A_2$

$\quad\quad H_2 = K_o + a_1 + a_2$

For an intravascular bolus injection of one unit of protein at time $t=0$, i.e. $\bar{F}(s)=1$, the first equation (A21) may then be written:

$$\bar{P}_b(s) = \frac{(s+a_1)(s+a_2)}{(s+k_1)(s+k_2)(s+k_3)} = \frac{P_1}{s+k_1} + \frac{P_2}{s+k_2} + \frac{P_3}{s+k_3} =$$

$$= \frac{P_1(s+k_2)(s+k_3) + P_2(s+k_1)(s+k_3) + P_3(s+k_1)(s+k_2)}{(s+k_1)(s+k_2)(s+k_3)} \tag{A23}$$

Again, the numerators in equation (A23) must be equal, also for special values of s. Chosing respectively the values $s=-k_1$, $s=-k_2$ and $s=-k_3$ one finds:

$$P_1(k_2-k_1)(k_3-k_1) = (a_1-k_1)(a_2-k_2) \; ; \; P_1 = \frac{(a_1-k_1)(a_2-k_2)}{(k_2-k_1)(k_3-k_1)}$$

$$P_2(k_1-k_2)(k_3-k_2) = (a_1-k_2)(a_2-k_2) \; ; \; P_2 = \frac{(a_1-k_2)(a_2-k_2)}{(k_1-k_2)(k_3-k_2)} \tag{A24}$$

$$P_3(k_1-k_3)(k_2-k_3) = (a_1-k_3)(a_2-k_3) \; ; \; P_3 = \frac{(a_1-k_3)(a_2-k_3)}{(k_1-k_3)(k_2-k_3)}$$

From equation (A23) it follows that P(t) is given by:

$$P(t) = P_1 e^{-k_1 t} + P_2 e^{-k_2 t} + P_3 e^{-k_3 t} \tag{A25}$$

The parameters P_1, P_2, P_3, k_1, k_2 and k_3 of this tri-exponential disappearance curve can be calculated from equations (A21), (A22) and (A24).

Inserting equation (A23) into equation (A21) one obtains:

$$\bar{E}_{1b}(s) = \frac{A_1 s + B_1}{(s+k_1)(s+k_2)(s+k_3)} = \frac{R_1}{s+k_1} + \frac{R_2}{s+k_2} + \frac{R_3}{s+k_3} \tag{A26}$$

From the equality of the numerators of these expressions for $s=-k_1$ and $s=-k_2$ one obtains:

$$R_1(k_2-k_1)(k_3-k_1) = -A_1 k_1 + B_1 \quad ; \quad R_1 = \frac{B_1 - A_1 k_1}{(k_2-k_1)(k_3-k_1)}$$

$$\tag{A27}$$

$$R_2(k_1-k_2)(k_3-k_2) = -A_1 k_2 + B_1 \quad ; \quad R_2 = \frac{B_1 - A_1 k_2}{(k_1-k_2)(k_3-k_2)}$$

$$R_1 + R_2 + R_3 = 0$$

For $\bar{E}_{2b}(s) = \frac{S_1}{s+k_1} + \frac{S_2}{s+k_2} + \frac{S_3}{s+k_3}$, analogous expressions are found with A_1, B_1 replaced by A_2, B_2.

We now consider the reverse problem, i.e. calculation of the model parameters in Fig. A2 from the parameters P_1, P_2, P_3, k_1, k_2, k_3, R_1, R_2, R_3, S_1, S_2 and S_3 determined from the disappearance curves $P_b(t)$, $E_{1b}(t)$ and $E_{2b}(t)$. From equations (A19) and (A25) one obtains:

$$-[\frac{d}{dt} P_b(t)]_{t=0} = K_o = P_1 k_1 + P_2 k_2 + P_3 k_3 \tag{A28}$$

Equating the numerators of equation (A23) it is found that

$$a_{1,2} = \tfrac{1}{2}(H_1 \pm \sqrt{H_1^2 - 4H_2}) \tag{A29}$$

with $H_1 = P_1(k_2+k_3) + P_2(k_1+k_3) + P_3(k_1+k_2)$

$H_2 = P_1 k_2 k_3 + P_2 k_1 k_3 + P_3 k_1 k_2$

Equating the denumerators of equation (A23) and the first equation (A21) after inserting $s=-a_1$ and $s=-a_2$ one finds:

$$(k_1-a_1)(k_2-a_1)(k_3-a_1) = (ERR_1 \cdot A_1 + ERR_2 \cdot A_2)a_1 - ERR_1 \cdot B_1 - ERR_2 \cdot B_2$$

$$(k_1-a_2)(k_2-a_2)(k_3-a_2) = (ERR_1 \cdot A_1 + ERR_2 \cdot A_2)a_2 - ERR_1 \cdot B_1 - ERR_2 \cdot B_2$$

or

$$ERR_1 \cdot A_1 + ERR_2 \cdot A_2 = \frac{(k_1-a_2)(k_2-a_2)(k_3-a_2)-(k_1-a_1)(k_2-a_1)(k_3-a_1)}{a_2 - a_1}$$

$$ERR_1 \cdot B_1 + ERR_2 \cdot B_2 = \frac{a_1(k_1-a_2)(k_2-a_2)(k_3-a_2)-a_2(k_1-a_1)(k_2-a_1)(k_3-a_1)}{a_2 - a_1}$$

$$(A30)$$

Equating the numerators of equation (A26) for $\overline{E}_{1b}$ and $\overline{E}_{2b}$, explicit expressions for A_1, A_2, B_1 and B_2 are obtained:

$$TER_1 = A_1 = R_1(k_2+k_3) + R_2(k_1+k_3) + R_3(k_1+k_2)$$

$$B_1 = R_1k_2k_3 + R_2k_1k_3 + R_3k_1k_2$$

$$(A31)$$

$$TER_2 = A_2 = S_1(k_2+k_3) + S_2(k_1+k_3) + S_3(k_1+k_2)$$

$$B_2 = S_1k_2k_3 + S_2k_1k_3 + S_3k_1k_2$$

Values of TER_1, TER_2, ERR_1 and ERR_2 can be calculated from equations (A30) and (A31) and FCR is calculated from equation (A28). Equating the values of H_1 and H_2 in equations (A29) and (A21) and the values of B_1 and B_2 in equations (A31) and (A21) one may then calculate k_{e1}, k_{e2}, k_{12} and k_{21}.

Three-compartment mammillary model

The tri-phasic plasma disappearance curve

$$P_b(t) = P_1 e^{-k_1t} + P_2 e^{-k_2t} + P_3 e^{-k_3t} \; ; \; P_1+P_2+P_3 = 1 \quad (A32)$$

only contains 5 independent parameters which implies that only 5 model parameters can be determined in those cases where $E_{1b}(t)$ and $E_{2b}(t)$ cannot be separately measured. This means that the model presented in Fig. A2 has to be simplified considerably. A much-used version of such a simplified model is shown in Fig. A3.

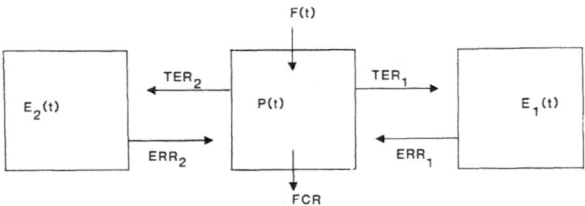

Fig. A.3.   Three-compartment mammillary system.

According to equation (A24) we have:

$$P_1 = \frac{(a_1-k_1)(a_2-k_2)}{(k_2-k_1)(k_3-k_1)} \; ; \; P_2 = \frac{(a_1-k_2)(a_2-k_2)}{(k_1-k_2)(k_3-k_2)} \; ; \; P_3 = 1-P_1-P_2$$

From equations (A21) and (A22) we find that in this case:

$$a_1 = K_1 = ERR_1 \; ; \; a_2 = K_2 = ERR_2$$

while k_1, k_2 and k_3 are the roots of the cubic equation:

$$s^3 + H_2 s^2 + H_1 s + H_o = 0$$

with $H_o = FCR.ERR_1.ERR_2$

$$H_1 = FCR(ERR_1+ERR_2) + TER_1.ERR_2 + TER_2.ERR_1 + ERR_1.ERR_2$$

$$H_2 = FCR + TER_1 + TER_2 + ERR_1 + ERR_2$$

The reverse problem of calculation of model parameters from P_1, P_2, P_3, k_1, k_2 and k_3 can besolved as follows. From equations (A21) and (A29) one finds:

$$ERR_1 = a_1 = \tfrac{1}{2}(H_1 + \sqrt{H_1^2 - 4H_2})$$

$$ERR_2 = a_2 = \tfrac{1}{2}(H_1 - \sqrt{H_1^2 - 4H_2})$$

with $H_1 = P_1(k_2+k_3) + P_2(k_1+k_3) + P_3(k_1+k_2)$

$$H_2 = P_1 k_2 k_3 + P_2 k_1 k_3 + P_3 k_1 k_2$$

From equation (A30) one finds:

$$TER_1 = (k_1-ERR_1)(k_2-ERR_1)(k_3-ERR_1)/(ERR_1^2-ERR_1.ERR_2)$$

$$TER_2 = (k_1-ERR_2)(k_2-ERR_2)(k_3-ERR_2)/(ERR_2{}^2-ERR_1 \cdot ERR_2)$$

From equation (A28) one finds

$$FCR = P_1k_1 + P_2k_2 + P_3k_3 - TER_1 - TER_2$$

A simple expression for FCR can also be given for models with only intravascular elimination of protein. Complete elimination of one unit of intravascularly injected protein in that case implies:

$$1 = FCR \cdot \int_0^t P(\tau)d\tau$$

or using equation (A32) for P(t):

$$FCR = 1/\int_0^\infty P(\tau)d\tau = 1/(P_1/k_1+P_2/k_2+P_3/k_3)$$

Nosslin's integral method

From equation (4.2) it follows that a steady-state input $F(t)=F_s$ in plasma starting at t=0 will result in the following expression for the plasma protein pool:

$$P(t) = F_s \int_0^t P_b(t-\tau)d\tau = F_s \cdot -\int_t^0 P_b(\xi)d\xi = F_s \int_0^t P_b(\tau)d\tau$$

where $P_b(t)$ is the plasma response curve to an intravascular bolus injection of one unit of protein. Similarly, one finds:

$$E(t) = F_s \int_0^t E_b(\tau)d\tau$$

where $E_b(t)$ is the extravascular response curve to an intravascular bolus injection of one unit of protein. For $t \to \infty$, P(t) and E(t) will reach their steady:state values P_s and E_s:

$$(E/P)_s = \int_0^\infty E_b(\tau)d\tau/\int_0^\infty P_b(\tau)d\tau = (\int_0^\infty T_b(\tau)d\tau/\int_0^\infty P_b(\tau)d\tau)-1$$

$$(A33)$$

The intravascularly injected unit of protein will eventually be eliminated:

$$1 \quad = FCR \int_o^\infty P_b(\tau)d\tau + k_e \int_o^\infty E_b(\tau)d\tau$$

$$= FCR \int_o^\infty P_b(\tau)d\tau + k_e \cdot (E/P)_s \int_o^\infty P_b(\tau)d\tau \qquad (A34)$$

(A33)

$$k_{tot} = FCR + k_e \cdot (E/P)_s = 1 / \int_o^\infty P_b(\tau)d\tau$$

If it is now assumed that the elimination of protein occurs intravascularly one has:

$$1 = P_b(t) + E_b(t) + FCR. \int_o^t P_b(\tau)d\tau$$

$$or \quad E_b(t) = 1 - FCR. \int_o^t P_b(\tau)d\tau - P_b(t)$$

$$= FCR. \int_t^\infty P_b(\tau)d\tau - P_b(t)$$

Integrating this integration we obtain:

$$\int_o^\infty E_b(\tau)d\tau = FCR. \int_o^\infty dt \int_t^\infty P_b(\tau)d\tau - \int_o^\infty P_b(\tau)d\tau$$

or after partial integration:

$$\int_o^\infty E_b(\tau)d\tau = FCR. \int_o^\infty \tau \, P_b(\tau)d\tau - \int_o^\infty P_b(\tau)d\tau$$

Combining this equation with equations (A33) and (A34) one obtains:

$$(E/P)_s = \int_o^\infty \tau \, P_b(\tau)d\tau / (\int_o^\infty P_b(\tau)d\tau)^2 - 1 \qquad (A35)$$

Effect of sudden depletion of the plasma protein pool and sudden changes in the rate of protein synthesis

The changes in time of the plasma protein pool P(t) and the extravascular protein pool $E(t)$ in a general two-compartment model can be written:

$$\frac{d}{dt} P(t) = -K_p \cdot P(t) + ERR \cdot E(t) + F(t) \quad ; \quad K_p = FCR + TER$$

$$\frac{d}{dt} E(t) = -K_e \cdot E(t) + TER \cdot P(t) \quad\quad ; \quad K_E = k_e + ERR$$

If the system is in a steady state one has:

$$F(t) = F_s \quad ; \quad E_s = \frac{TER}{K_E} P_s \quad ; \quad (K_p - \frac{ERR \cdot TER}{K_E}) P_s = F_s$$

From these equations it may be verified that the changes in time of $\Delta P = P_s - P$ and $\Delta E = E_s - E$ can be written as

$$\frac{d}{dt} \Delta P = -K_p \cdot \Delta P + ERR \cdot \Delta E$$

$$\frac{d}{dt} \Delta E = -K_E \cdot \Delta E + TER \cdot \Delta P$$

$$(A36)$$

If the plasma pool is suddenly depleted at time $t=0$, these equators must be solved for the conditions $\Delta P(t=0) = P_s$ and $\Delta E(t=0) = 0$. This implies that the solution of equations (A36) are identical to the response curves on an intravascular bolus of P_s units of protein at time $t=0$.

We now consider a sudden change in the rate of protein entrance into plasma:

$$t \leq 0 \quad F(t) = F_s$$

$$t > 0 \quad F(t) = F_1$$

The plasma protein pool $P(t)$ can be calculated from the expression:

$$P(t) = \int_{-\infty}^{t} F(\tau) \, P_b(t-\tau) \, d\tau \quad \text{with} \quad P_b(t) = P_1 e^{-k_1 t} + P_2 e^{-k_2 t}$$

For $t \leq 0$ one obtains:

$$P(t) = F_s \int_{-\infty}^{t} P_b(t-\tau) \, d\tau = F_s \int_{0}^{\infty} P_b(\tau) \, d\tau = F_s (\frac{P_1}{k_1} + \frac{P_2}{k_2}) = P_s$$

For $t > 0$ one obtains:

$$P(t) = F_s \int_{-\infty}^{0} P_b(t-\tau) d\tau + F_1 \int_{0}^{t} P_b(t-\tau) d\tau$$

$$= F_s \int_{t}^{\infty} P_b(\tau) d\tau + F_1 \int_{0}^{t} P_b(\tau) d\tau$$

$$= F_s(\frac{P_1}{k_1} e^{-k_1 t} + \frac{P_2}{k_2} e^{-k_2 t}) + F_1(\frac{P_1}{k_1} + \frac{P_2}{k_2} - \frac{P_1}{k_1} e^{-k_1 t} - \frac{P_2}{k_2} e^{-k_2 t})$$

This expression for P(t) can be written as

$$\Delta P(t) = P_s - P(t) = Q_1 + Q_2 - Q_1 e^{-k_1 t} - Q_2 e^{-k_2 t}$$

$$\text{with } Q_1 = \Delta F \cdot P_1/k_1 \; ; \; Q_2 = \Delta F \cdot P_2/k_2 \; ; \; \Delta F = F_s - F_1$$

(A37)

REFERENCES

1. Abildgaard CF, Simone JV, Corrigan JJ, Seeler RA, Edelstein G, Vanderheiden J, Schulman J: Treatment of hemophilia with glycine-precipitated factor VIII. New Eng J Med 275, 471-475, 1966.
2. Adams RD: Diseases of muscle. Harper and Row Publ, New York,1975,3rd ed.
3. Adelson E, Rheingold JJ, Parker O, Steiner M, Kirby JC: The survival of factor VIII (antihemophilic globulin) and factor IX (plasma thromboplastin component) in normal humans. J Clin Invest 42, 1040-1047, 1963.
4. Afonso S, Rowe GG, Lugo JE, Crumpton CW: Left ventricle heat production in intact anesthetized dogs. Am J Physiol 208, 946-953, 1965.
5. Agress CM, Jacobs HJ, Glassner HF, Lederer MA, Clark WG, Wroblewski F, Karmen A, La Due JS: Serum transaminase levels in experimental myocardial infarction. Circulation 11, 711-713, 1955.
6. Alderman EL, Matlof HJ, Shumway NE, Harrison D: Evaluation of enzyme testing for the detection of myocardial infarction following direct coronary surgery. Circulation 48, 135-140, 1973.
7. Allsopp D, Bailey PJ, Higgins TJC: The effects of incubation conditions on enzyme release from anoxic heart cell cultures. J Mol Cell Card 12: 701-714, 1980.
8. Alper AC, Freeman T, Waldenström J: The metabolism of gamma globulins in myeloma and allied conditions. J Clin Invest 42, 1858-1868, 1963.
9. Alper CA, Peters JH, Birtsch AG, Gardner FH: Haptoglobin synthesis I. In vivo studies of the production of haptoglobin, fibrinogen and alpha-globulin by the canine liver. J Clin Invest 44, 574-581, 1965.
10. Alper CA: Complement. In: Structure and function of plasma proteins. AC Allison (Ed), Plenum Press, London, 1, 1974, 195-222.
11. Amelung D: Untersuchungen zur Grösze der Eliminationsgeschwindigkeit von Fermenten aus dem Kaninchenserum. Hoppe-Seylers Z Physiol Chem 318, 219-228, 1960.
12. Amelung D: Enzymelimination aus dem Plasma. In: Praktische Enzymologie. Schmidt FW (Ed), Bern, Huber HT, 1968, 149-162.
13. Amery A, Roeber G, Vermeulen HJ, Verstraete M: Single-blind randomized multicentre trial comparing heparin and streptokinase treatment in recent myocardial infarction. Acta Med Scand, Suppl 1969, 505,1-35.
14. Andersen SB, Glemert J, Wallevik K: Gamma globulin turnover and intestinal degradation of gamma globulin in the dog. J Clin Invest 42, 1873-1881, 1963.
15. Andersen SB: Metabolism of human gamma-globulin. Oxford, Blackwell Scientific Publ, 1964.
16. Anderson MC, Schiller WR: Microcirculatory dynamics in the normal and inflamed pancreas. Am J Surg 115, 118-127, 1968.
17. Anderson CB, Codd JE, Graff RJ, Gregory JG, Groce MA, Newton WT: Serum lactic dehydrogenase and human renal allograft failure. Surgery 77, 674-679, 1975.
18. Appert AR, Dimbiglu M, Pairent FW, Howard JM: The disappearance of intravenously injected pancreatic enzymes. Surg Gynecol Obstet 127, 1281-1287, 1968.
19. Arnesen H, Fagerhol MK: Alpha-2-macroglobulin, alpha-1-antitrypsin and antithrombin III in plasma and serum during fibrinolytic therapy with urokinase. Scand J Clin Lab Clin Invest 29, 259-263, 1972.
20. Aronson KF, Ekelund G, Kindmark CO, Laurell CB: Sequential changes of plasma proteins after surgical trauma. Scand J Clin Lab Invest 29, Suppl 124, 127-136, 1972.

21. Arts T, Reneman RS, Veenstra PC: A model of the mechanics of the left ventricle. Ann Biomed Engin 7, 299-318, 1979.
22. Arts T, Reneman RS: Measurement of deformation of canine epicardium in vivo during cardiac cycle. Am J Physiol 239, H432-H437, 1980.
23. Ashwell G, Morell AG: The role of surface carbohydrates in the hepatic recognition and transport of circulating glycoproteins. Adv Enzymol 41, 99-127, 1974.
24. Aukland K, Nicolaysen G: Interstitial fluid volume; local regulatory mechanisms. Physiol Rev 61, 556-643, 1981.
25. Austen DEG, Rizza CR: The biochemistry of blood clotting factors. In: Structure and function of plasma proteins. AC Allison (Ed), Plenum Press, London, 1974, 169-194.
26. Awai M, Brown EB: Studies of the metabolism of I-131-labeled human transferrin. J Lab Clin Med 61, 363-396. 1963.
27. Awwad HK, El Sheraky AS, Helmi SA, Shetaiwy SK, Potchen EJ: The relationship between serum albumin and sulfate synthesis. A method for the measurement of synthesis of liver-produced plasma proteins using 35 S-1-Cystine. J Biol Chem 245, 469-476, 1970.
28. Baele G, Mussche M, Vermeire P: Serum fibrin/fibrinogen degradation products in acute myocardial infarction. Lancet 1,689-690,1972.
29. Bär U, Ohlendorf S: Studien zur Enzymelimination I. Halbwertzeiten einiger Zellenzyme beim Menschen. Klin Wschr 48, 776-780, 1970.
30. Bär U, Friedel R, Heine H, Mayer D, Ohlendorf S, Schmidt FW, Trautschold J: Studies on enzyme elimination III. Distribution, transport and elimination of cell enzymes in the extra cellular space. Enzyme 14: 133-156, 1972/1973.
31. Barlow CH, Chance B: Ischemic areas in perfused rat hearts: measurement by NADH fluorescence photography. Science 193, 909-910, 1967.
32. Barth WF, Wochner RD, Waldmann TA, Fahey JL: Metabolism of human gamma macroglobulins. J Clin Invest 43, 1036-1048, 1964.
33. Bartsch RC, McConnell EE, Imes GD, Schmidt JM: A review of exertional rhabdomyolysis in wild and domestic animals and man. Vet Pathol 14, 314-324, 1977.
34. Bauman A, Rothschild MA, Yalow RS, Berson SA: Distribution and metabolism of 131-I labeled human serum albumin in congestive heart failure with and without proteinuria. J Clin Invest 34, 1359-1368, 1955.
35. Baur HR, Steele BW, Freimesberger KF, Gobel FL: Serum myocardial creatine kinase (CK-MB) after coronary arterial bypass surgery. Am J Cardiol 44, 679-686, 1979.
36. Bear H, Blount SG: The response of the serum glutamic oxalacetic transaminase to open-heart operation. Am Heart J 60,867-875,1960.
37. Beeken WL, Volwiler W, Goldsworthy PD, Garby LE, Reynolds WE, Stogsdill R, Stemler RS: Studies of I-131-ablumin catabolism and distribution in normal young male adults. J Clin Invest 41, 1312-1333, 1962.
38. Benacerraf B, Biozzi G, Halpern BN, Stiffel C, Mouton D: Phagocytosis of heat-denatured human serum albumin labeled with 131-I and its use as a means of investigating liver blood flow. Br J Expl Pathol 38, 35-48, 1957.
39. Benamon-Djiane D, Drouet J, Cosson A, Blatrix C, Ménaché D, Josso F: Durée de vie chez l'homme de la prothrombine marquée par l'iode radioactif (131 I). Rev Franc Transfusion 11, 129-138, 1968.
40. Bendz R, Ström S, Olin C: CK-MB in serum and in heart and skeletal muscles in patients subjected to mitral valve replacement. Eur J Cardiol 12, 25-39, 1980.
41. Bennett RM, Kokocinski T: Lactoferrin turnover in man. Clin Sci 57, 453-460, 1979.

42. Bennhold H, Kallee E: Comparative studies on the half-life of I-131 labeled albumins and nonradioactive human serum albumin in a case of analbuminemia. J Clin Invest 38, 863-872, 1959.

43. Berenbom M, Chang PJ, Betz HE, Stowell RE: Chemical and enzymatic changes associated with mouse liver necrosis in vitro. Cancer Res 15, 1-5, 1955.

44. Berenbom M, Chang PJ, Stowell RE: Changes in mouse liver undergoing necrosis in vivo. Lab Invest 4, 315-323, 1955.

45. Berg A, Haralambie G: Changes in serum creatine kinase and hexose phosphate isomerase activity with exercise duration. Eur J Appl Physiol 39, 191-201, 1978.

46. Bergmeyer HV: Methoden der enzymatischen Analyse. Weinheim/ Bergsh, Verlag Chemie, 1974 Band I, 3 Auflage.

47. Berman M, Schoenfeld R: Invariants in experimental data on linear kinetics and the formulation of models. J Appl Physics 27,1361-1372,1956.

48. Berman M, Hall M, Levy RJ, Eisenberg S, Bilheimer DW, Phair RD, Goebel RH: Metabolism of apo B and apo C lipoproteins in man; kinetic studies in normal and hyperlipoproteinemic subjects. J Lipid Res 19, 38-56, 1978.

49. Berson SA, Yalow RS: The use of K-42 or P-32 labeled erythrocytes and I-131 tagged human serum albumin in simultaneous blood volume determinations. J Clin Invest 31, 572-580, 1952.

50. Berson SA, Yalow RS, Schreiber SS, Post J: Tracer experiments with I-131 labeled human serum albumin: distribution and degradation studies. J Clin Invest 32, 746-768, 1953.

51. Berson SA, Yalow RS: The distribution of I-131 labeled human serum albumin introduced into ascitic fluid: analysis of the kinetics of a three compartment catenary transfer system in man and speculations on possible sites of degradation. J Clin Invest 33, 377-387, 1954.

52. Berson SA: Blood volume in health and disease. Bull NY Acad Med 30, 750-776, 1954.

53. Berson SA,Yalow RS: Distribution and metabolism of 131-I labeled proteins in man. Fed Proc 13,135-145,1957.

54. Beutler E, Blume KG, Kaplan JC, Löhr GW, Ramot B, Valentine WN: International committee for standardisation in haematology: recommended methods for red-cell enzyme analysis. Br J Haematol 35, 331-340, 1977.

55. Bianchi R, Mariani G, Pilo A, Toni MG, Donato L: Short-term determination of plasma protein turnover by a two-tracer technique using plasma only or plasma and urine data. In: Protein Turnover. Ciba Foundation Symp 9 (new series) Amsterdam, Elsevier, 47-72, 1973.

56. Bianchi R, Mariani G, McFarlane AS: Plasma protein turnover. London, MacMillan Press Ltd, 1976.

57. Biggs RR: The turnover of factors II, VIII, IX and X in patients deficient in these factors. Thrombos Diathes Haemorrh 9 , suppl 13, 201-208, 1963.

58. Biggs R, Denson KWE: The fate of prothrombin and factors VIII, IX and X transfused to patients deficient in these factors. Br J Haemathol 9, 532-547, 1963.

59. Billah MM, Finean JB, Coleman R, Michell RH: Permeability characteristics of erythrocyte ghosts prepared under isotonic conditions by a glycol-induced osmotic lysis. Biochim Biophys Acta 465, 515-526, 1977.

60. Birke G, Liljedahl S-O, Plantin L-O, Wetterfors J: Albumin catabolism in burns and following surgical procedures. Acta Chir Scand 118, 353-366, 1959/1960.

61. Bleifeld W, Mathey D, Hanrath P, Buss H, Effert S: Infarct size estimated from serial serum creatine phosphokinase in relation to left ventricle dynamics. Circulation 55, 303-311, 1977.

62. Blombäck B, Carlson LA, Franzén S, Zetterqvist E: Turnover of 131-I-

labelled fibrinogen in man. Studies in normal subjects, in congenital coagulation factor deficiency states, in liver cirrhosis, in polycythemia Vera and in epidermolysis Bullosa. Acta Med Scand 179, 557-574, 1966.

63. Bloom AL: The biosynthesis of factor VIII. Clinics Haemat 8, 53-77, 1979.

64. Blum CB, Levy RJ, Eisenberg S, Hall M, Goebel RH, Berman M: High density lipoprotein metabolism in man. J Clin Invest 60, 795-807, 1977.

65. Bolooki H, Sommer L, Faraldo A, Ghahramani A, Slavin D, Kaiser GA: The significance of serum enzyme studies in patients undergoing direct coronary artery surgery. J Thorac Cardiovasc Surg 65, 863-868, 1973.

66. Bond JS: A comparison of the proteolytic susceptibility of several rat liver enzymes. Biochem Biophys Res Comm 43, 333-339, 1971.

67. Borchgrevink CF, Egeberg O, Pool JG, Skulason T, Stormorken H, Waaler B: A study of a case of congenital hypoprothrombinaemia. Br J Haematol 5, 294-300, 1959.

68. Borchgrevink CF, Owren PA: Surgery in a patient with factor V (proaccelerin) deficiency. Acta Med Scand 170, 743-746, 1961.

69. Böttiger LE, Molin L: Turnover of 131-I and 125-I-labelled haptoglobin in man. Acta Med Scand 184, 187-190, 1968.

70. Bowie EJW, Thompson JH, Didisheim P, Owen CA: Disappearance rates of coagulation factors: transfusion studies in factor deficient patients. Transfusion 7, 174-184, 1967.

71. Brace RA, Taylor AE, Guyton AC: Time course of lymph protein concentration in the dog. Microvasc Res 14, 243-249, 1977.

72. Brauer RW: Liver circulation and function. Physiol Rev 43, 115-213, 1963.

73. Briem H, Helgason T, Gudmundsson TV: Long-term effect of clofibrate on albumin turnover and distribution in man. Acta Med Scand 203, 205-210, 1978.

74. Brightman MW, Klatzo J, Olsson Y, Reese TS: The blood-brain barrier to proteins under normal and pathological conditions. J Neurol Sci 10, 215-239, 1970.

75. Britten AFH: Congenital deficiency of factor XIII (fibrin-stabilizing factor). Am J Med 43, 751-761, 1967.

76. Brodsky J, Siegel NH, Kahn SB, Ross EM, Petkov G: Simultaneous fibrinogen and platelet survival with [75Se] selenomethionine in man. Studies in diseases with normal coagulation and in hepatocellular disease with abnormal coagulation. Br J Haematol 18, 341-355, 1970.

77. Brown RF: Compartmental system analysis; state of the art. IEEE Trans Biomed Eng, BME-27, 1-11, 1980.

78. Bruning PF, Loeliger EA: Prothrombal: a new concentrate of human prothrombin complex for clinical use. Br J Haematol 21, 377-398, 1971.

79. Burch GE, DePasquale NP: The hematocrit in patients with myocardial infarction. JAMA 180, 63-65, 1962.

80. Caen J, Yanotti S, Varangot J, Bernard J: Etude d'un cas d'hypoproconvertinémie vraie congénitale. Sang 30, 535-547, 1959.

81. Cailar C, Maille J-G, Jones W, Solymoss BC, Chabot M, Goulet C, Delva E, Grondin CM: MB-creatine kinase and the evaluation of myocardial injury following aorto-coronary bypass operation. Ann Thor Surg 29, 8-14, 1980.

82. Cain H, Assmann W: Bedeutung und Problematik enzymatischer Gewebs- und Serumbefunde beim frischen myokardinfarkt. Klin Wschr 38, 433-439, 1960.

83. Cairns JA, Missirilis E, Fallen EL: Myocardial infarction size from serial CPK: variability of CPK serum entry ratio with size and model of infarction. Circulation 58, 1143-1153, 1978.

84. Calvert, GD, James HM: Low-density lipoprotein turnover studies in man. Evaluation of the integrated rate equations method, use of a whole-body radioactivity counter, and the problem of partial denaturation. Clin Sci 56, 71-76, 1979.

85. Campbell RM, Cuthbertson DP, Matthews CM, Mc Farlane AS: Behaviour of 14C- and 131-I-labelled plasma proteins in the rat. Int J Appl Rad Isot 1, 66-84, 1956.

86. Carpenter CB, Ruddy S, Shehadeh I, Müller-Eberhard HJ, Merrill JP, Austen KF: Complement metabolism in man: hypercatabolism of the fourth (C4) and third (C3) components in patients with renal allograft rejection and hereditary angioedema (HAE). J Clin Invest 48, 1495-1505, 1969.

87. Cavalieri RR, McMahon FA, Castle JN: Preparation of 125-I-labeled human thyroxine-binding alpha globulin and its turnover in normal and hypothyroid subjects. J Clin Invest 56, 79-87, 1975.

88. Chapelle J-P, Heusghem C: Further heterogeneity demonstrated for serum creatine kinase isoenzyme MM. Clin Chem 26, 457-462, 1980.

89. Chapman BL: Correlation of mortality rate and serum enzymes in myocardial infarction. Br Heart J 33, 643-646, 1971.

90. Charlesworth JA, Williams DG, Sherington E, Lachmann PJ, Peters DK: Metabolic studies of the third component of complement and the glycine-rich beta glycoprotein in patients with hypocomplementemia. J Clin Invest 53, 1578-1587, 1974.

91. Charlesworth JA, Williams DG, Sherington E, Peters DK: Metabolism of the third component of complement (C3) in normal human subjects. Clin Sci Mol Med 46, 223-229, 1974.

92. Charlesworth JA, Scott DM, Pussell, BA, Peters DK: Metabolism of human beta 1H: studies in man and experimental animals. Clin Exp Immunol 38, 397-404, 1979.

93. Chen YH, Reeve EB: Some factors influencing metabolism and distribution of fibrinogen in man and rabbits. Thromb Haemostas (Stuttg) 37, 243-252, 1977.

94. Clark GL, Robison AK, Gnepp DR, Roberts R, Sobel BE: Effects of lymphatic transport of enzyme on plasma creatine kinase time-activity curves after myocardial infarction in dogs. Circ Res 43, 162-169, 1978.

95. Clubb JS, Neale FC, Posen S: The behavior of infused human placental alkaline phosphatase in human subjects. J Lab Clin Med 66, 493-507, 1965.

96. Codd JE, Kaiser GC, Wiens RD, Barner HB, Willman VL: Myocardial injury and bypass grafting. Value of serum enzymes in diagnosis. J Thorac Cardiovasc Surg 70, 489-494, 1975.

97. Codd JE, Sullivan RG, Weins RD, Barner HB, Kaiser GC, Willman VL: Myocardial injury following myocardial revascularization. Detection by isoenzyme analysis. Circulation 56, suppl 2, II 49-II 53, 1977.

98. Cohen S, Holloway RC, Mathews C, McFarlane AS: Distribution and elimination of 131-I- and 14C-labelled plasma proteins in the rabbit. Biochem J 62, 143-154, 1956.

99. Cohen S, Freeman T: Metabolic heterogeneity of human gamma-globulin. Biochem J 76, 475-487, 1960.

100. Cohen S, Freeman T, McFarlane AS: Metabolism of 131-I labeled human albumin. Clin Sci 20, 161-170, 1961.

101. Coles GA, Peters DK, Jones JH: Albumin metabolism in chronic renal failure. Clin Sci 39, 423-435, 1970.

102. Collen D, Tytgat GN, Claeys H, Piessens R: Metabolism and distribution of fibrinogen. I. Fibrinogen turnover in physiological conditions in humans. Br J Haematol 22, 681-700, 1972.

103. Collen D, Tytgat G, Claeys H, Verstraete M, Wallén P: Metabolism of plasminogen in healthy subjects: Effect of tranexamic acid. J Clin Invest 51, 1310-1318, 1972.

104. Collen D, Schetz J, de Cock F, Holmer E, Verstraete M: Metabolism of antithrombin III (heparin cofactor) in man - effects of venous thrombosis and of heparin administration. Eur J Clin Invest 7, 27-35, 1977.

105. Collen D, Semeraro N, Tricot JP, Vermijlen J: Turnover of fibrinogen, plasminogen and prothrombin during exercise in man. J Appl Physiol 42, 865-873, 1977.
106. Colowick SP, Kaplan MO: Methods in Enzymology. 80, part C. Proteolytic enzymes. L. Lorand (Ed), New York, 1981.
107. Conley CL, Russell RP, Thomas CB, Tumulty PA: Hematocrit values in coronary artery disease. Arch Int Med 113, 170-176, 1964.
108. Conti VR, Bertranou EG, Blackstone EH, Kirklin JW, Digerness SB: Cold cardioplegia versus hypothermia for myocardial protection. Randomized clinical study. J Thorac Cardiovasc Surg 76, 577-589, 1978.
109. Conway TP, Morgan WT, Liem HH, Müller-Eberhard U: Catabolism of photo-oxidized and desialylated hemopexin in the rabbit. J Biol Chem 250, 3067-3073, 1975.
110. Coodley EL: Diagnostic enzymology. Philadelphia, Lea and Febiger, 1970.
112. Curran PF, Taylor AE, Solomon AK: Tracer diffusion and unidirectional flows. Biophys J 7, 879-901, 1967.
111. Coward WA, Sawyer MB: Whole-body albumin mass and distribution in rats fed on low protein diets. Br J Nutr 37,127-134,1977.
113. Dalgaard JB: Serum phosphatase after transfusion of phosphate-rich blood to normal dogs. Acta Physiol Scand 22, 193-199, 1951.
114. DaLuz PL, Shubin H, Weil MH, Jacobson E, Stein L: Pulmonary edema related to changes in colloid osmotic and pulmonary artery wedge pressure in patients after acute myocardial infarction. Circulation 51, 350-357, 1975.
115. Darcy DA: Response of a serum glycoprotein to tissue injury and necrosis. I. The response to necrosis, hyperplasia and tumour growth. Br J Exp Pathol 51, 281-293, 1964.
116. Davids HA, Hermens WT, Hollaar L, Van der Laarse A, Huysmans HA: Extent of myocardial damage after open-heart surgery assessed from serial plasma enzyme levels in either of two periods (1975-1980). Br Heart J 47,167-172 ,1982.
117. Davidson E, Tomlin S: The levels of the plasma coagulation factors in the post-operative period. Thromb Diath Haemorrh 10, 81-87, 1963.
118. Davies JWL, Forsberg K, Liljedahl S-O, Martensson O, Reizenstein P: The effect of anticoagulants on postoperative fibrinogen metabolism. Acta Med Scand 194, 277-283, 1973.
119. Dawson DM: Efflux of enzymes from chicken muscle. Biochim Biophys Acta 113, 144-157, 1966.
120. Dawson DM, Alper CA, Seidman J, Mendelsohn J: Measurement of serum turnover rates. Ann Int Med 70, 799-805, 1969.
121. Day JF, Thorpe SR, Baynes JW: Nonenzymatically glucosylated albumin. In vitro preparation and isolation from normal human serum. J Biol Chem 254, 595-597, 1979.
122. Decker RS, Wildenthal K: Lysosomal alterations in hypoxic and reoxygenated hearts. I. Ultrastructural and cytochemical changes. Am J Pathol 98, 425-444, 1980.
123. Decker RS, Pool AR, Crie JS, Dingle JT, Wildenthal K: Lysosomal alterations in hypoxic and reoxygenated hearts II. Immunohistochemical and biochemical changes in cathepsin D. Am J Pathol 98, 445-456, 1980.
124. DeDuve CR, Beaufay H: Influences of ischemia on the state of some bound enzymes in rat liver. Biochem J 73, 610-616, 1959.
125. De Duve C: General properties of lysosomes. In: Ciba Found Symp Lysosomes. AVS De Reuck,MP Cameron (eds.),London,1963.
126. De Groot SR, Mazur P: Non-equilibrium thermodynamics. North-Holland Publ Cy, Amsterdam,1969.
127. Dehlinger PJ, Schimke RT: Effect of size on the relative rate of degrada-

tion of rat liver soluble proteins. Biochem Biophys Res Comm 40, 1473-1480, 1970.

128. De Leiris J, Feuvray D: Morphological correlates of myocardial enzyme release. In: Enzymes in cardiology. DJ Hearse, J de Leiris (Eds.), New York, John Wiley & Sons, 1979, 445-460.

129. Déleze J: The recovery of resting potential and input resistance in sheep heart injured by knife or laser. J Physiol 208, 547-562, 1970.

130. DeLuca A, Ingwall JS, Bittl JA: Biochemical response of myocardial cells in culture to oxygen and glucose deprivation. Biochem Biophys Res Comm 59, 749-756, 1974.

131. Delva E, Maillé J-G, Solymoss BC, Chabot M, Grondin C, Bourassa MG: Evaluation of myocardial damage during coronary artery grafting with serial determinations of serum CPK - MB isoenzyme. J Thorac Cardiovasc Surg 75, 467-475, 1978.

132. Demos MA, Gitin EL, Kager LJ: Exercise myoglobinemia and actue exertional rhabdomyolysis. Arch Intern Med 134, 669-673, 1974.

133. De Ritis F, Coltori M, Giusti G: Attivita transaminasica del sero umano nell' epatite virale. Minerva Medica 1, 1207-1209, 1955.

134. Dice JF, Goldberg AL: A statistical analysis of the relationship between degradative rates and molecular weights of proteins. Arch Biochem Biophys 170, 213-219, 1975.

135. Dike GWR, Griffiths D, Bidwell E, Snape TJ, Rizza CR: A factor VII concentrate for therapeutic use. Br J Haematol 45, 107-118, 1980.

136. Di Scipio RG, Hermodson MA, Yates SG, Davie EW: A comparison of human prothrombin, factor IX (Christmas factor), factor X (stuart factor) and protein S. Biochemistry 16, 698-706, 1977.

137. Dobryszycka W, Zeineh R, Ebroon E, Kukral JC: Metabolism of plasma proteins in injury states II. Incorporation of 14C glucosamine and 35S methionine into human and canine haptoglobin. Clin Sci 36, 231-240, 1969.

138. Dodds WJ. Packham MA, Rowsell HC, Mustard JF: Factor VII survival and turnover in dogs. Am J Physiol 213, 36-42, 1967.

139. Donato L: Round table on applications of tracer theory to protein turnover studies. In: Labeled proteins in tracer studies. L Donato, G Milhaud, J Sirchis (eds), Euratom, Brussels, 1966, 375-408.

140. Dowell RT: Transmural citrate synthase and lactate dehydrogenase levels in hypertrophied rat left ventricle. Proc Soc Exp Biol Med 158, 599-603, 1978.

141. Dubach VC, Schmidt V: Enzymology of human kidney. Enzym Biol Clin 11, 32-51, 1970.

142. Dunn M, Martins J, Reissmann KR: The disappearance rate of glutamic transaminase from the circulation and its distribution in the body's fluid compartments and secretions. J Lab Clin Med 51, 259-265, 1958.

143. Dykes PW, Davies JWL, Ricketts CR, Stanworth DR: The effect of plasma concentration on the catabolic rate of human serum albumin. In: Labelled proteins in tracer studies. L Donato, G Milhaud, J Sirchis (Eds), Brussels, Euratom, 1966, 113-124.

144. Egdahl RH: Mechanism of blood enzyme changes following the production of experimental pancreatitis. Ann Surg 148, 389-400, 1958.

145. Egeberg O: Changes in the coagulation system following major surgical operations. Acta Med Scand 171, 679-685, 1962

146. Engeset A, Aas M, Olszewsky W, Sokolowski J: Time of exchange of 131-I labeled albumin between plasma and peripheral lymph in man. Lymphology 12, 77-80, 1979.

147. Farrow SP, Baar S: The metabolism of alpha 2-macroglobulin in mildly burned patients. Clin Chim Acta 46, 39-48, 1973.

148. Fellenberg R, Eppenberger H, Richterich R, Aebi H: Das glykolytische En-

zymmuster von Leber, Niere, Skeletmuskel, Herzmuskel und Grosshirn bei Ratte und Maus. Biochem Z 336,334-350,1962.

149. Figueras J, Weil MH: Increases in plasma oncotic pressure during acute cardiogenic pulmonary edema. Circulation 55, 195-199, 1977.

150. Figueras J, Weil MH: Blood volume prior to and following treatment of acute cardiogenic pulmonary edema. Circulation 57, 349-355, 1978.

151. Fischbein M, Hare C, Gissen SA, Spadaro J, MacLean D, Maroko PR: Identification and quantification of histochemical border zones during the evolution of myocardial infarction in the rat. Cardiovasc Res 14, 41-49, 1980.

152. Fitts DD: Nonequilibrium thermodynamics. A phenomenological theory of irreversible processes in fluid systems. McGraw-Hill Book Cy,New York, 1962.

153. Fjeld NB, Kluge TH, Stokke KT, Skrede S: The effect of generalized hypoxia upon flow and composition of cardiac lymph in the dog. Eur J Clin Invest 6,255-259,1976.

154. Fleisher GA, Wakim KG: The fate of enzymes in body fluids - an experimental study I. Disappearance rates of glutamic - pyruvic transaminase under various conditions. J Lab Clin Med 61, 76-85, 1963.

155. Fleisher GA, Wakim KG: The fate of enzymes in body fluids - an experimental study III. Disappearance rates of glutamic-oxalacetic transaminase II under various conditions. J Lab Clin Med 61, 98-106, 1963.

156. Follette DM, Mulder DG, Maloney JV, Buckberg GD: Advantages of blood cardioplegia over continuous coronary perfusion or intermittent ischemia. Experimental and clinical study. J Thorac Cardiovasc Surg 76, 604-617, 1978.

157. Forsberg K, Torngren S: Deep venous thrombosis and multiple regression analysis of the influence from various clinical factors on the fibrinogen half life in surgical patients, using 125-I fibrinogen. Thromb Res 1,235-244,1977.

158. Freeman T, Gordon AH, Humphrey JH: Distinction between catabolism of native and denatured proteins by the isolated perfused liver after carbon loading. Br J Exptl Pathol 39, 459-471, 1958.

159. Freeman T: The biological behaviour of normal and denatured human plasma albumin. Clin Chim Acta 4, 788-792, 1959.

160. Freeman T, Matthews CME, McFarlane AS, Bennhold H, Kallee E: Albumin labelled with Iodine-131 in an analbuminaemic subject. Nature 183, 606, 1959.

161. Freeman T: Haptoglobin metabolism in relation to red cell destruction. In: Protides of the biological fluids 12, Amsterdam, Elsevier, 1964, 344-352.

162. Freeman T: Gamma globulin metabolism in normal humans and in patients. Ser Hemat 4, 76-86, 1965.

163. Freeman S, Cheng YP: The effect of jaundiced blood upon normal dogs, with special reference to the serum phosphatase. J Biol Chem 123, 239-246, 1938.

164. Frick PG: Studies on the turnover rate of stable prothrombin conversion factor in man. Acta haemat 19, 20-29, 1958.

165. Friedel R, Bode R, Trautschold J: Verteilung heterologer, homologer und autologer Enzyme nach intravenöser Injektion. Verteilung und Transport von Zellenzymen im extrazellulären Raum, III. Mitteilung. J Clin Chem Clin Biochem 14, 129-136, 1976

166. Friedel R, Diederichs F, Lindena J: Release and extracellular turnover of cellular enzymes. In: Advances in clinical enzymology. E Schmidt, FW Schmidt, J Trautschold, R Friedel (Eds), Basel, Karger S, 1979, 70-105.

167. Gebhard MM, Denkhaus H, Sakai K, Spieckermann PG: Energy metabolism and

enzyme release. J Mol Med 2: 271-283, 1977.

168. Getz GS, Hay RV: The formation and metabolism of plasma lipoproteins. In: The biochemistry of atherosclerosis. AM Scanu (ed),New York,1979,151-188.

169. Giesen J, Kammermeier H: Relationship of phosphorylation potential and oxygen consumption in isolated perfused hearts. J Mol Cell Cardiol 12, 891-907, 1980.

170. Gitlin D: Distribution dynamics of circulating and extravascular I 131 plasma proteins. Ann New York Acad Sci 70, 122-136, 1957.

171. Grotte G: Passage of dextran molecules across the blood-lymph barrier. Acta Chir Scand Suppl 211, 1-84, 1956.

172. Gollnick PD, Armstrong RB, Saubert JV, Piehl K, Saltin B: Enzyme activity and fiber composition in skeletal muscle of untrained and trained men. J Appl Physiol 33, 312-319, 1972.

173. Gordon AH: The rates of catabolism of rat transferrin in vivo and by the perfused rat liver. Protides of the Biological Fluids 10, 71-73, 1963.

174. Gray RJ, Harris WS, Shah PK, Miyamoto ATM, Matloff JM, Swan HJC: Coronary sinus blood flow and sampling for detection of unrecognized myocardial ischemia and injury. Circulation 56, Suppl 2, II 58-II 61, 1977.

175. Gray RJ, Shell WE, Conklin C, Ganz W, Shah PK, Miyamoto AT, Matloff JM, Swan HJC: Quantification of myocardial injury during coronary artery bypass graft. Circulation 58, suppl 1, 1-38/1-42, 1978.

176. Green D, Crews MC: Factor VIII labeled with radioiodine; preparation and metabolic studies. J Lab Clin Med 78, 840-841, 1971.

177. Grice HC, Barth ML, Cornish HH, Foster GF, Gray RH: Correlation between serum enzymes, isoenzyme patterns and histologically detectable organ damage. Fd Cosmet Toxicol 9, 847-855, 1971.

178. Grossman J, Yalow AA, Weston RE: Albumin degradation and synthesis as influenced by hydrocortison, corticotropin and infection. Metabolism 9, 528-550, 1960.

179. Gudbjarnason S, Cowan C, Braasch W, Bing RJ: Changes in enzyme pattern of infarcted heart muscle during tissue repair. Cardiologia 51, 148-159, 1967.

180. Guder WG, Habicht A, Kleissl J, Schmidt U, Wieland OH: The diagnostic significance of liver cell inhomogeneity: serum enzymes in patients with central liver necrosis and the distribution of glutamate dehydrogenase in normal human liver. Z Klin Chem Klin Biochem 13,311-318,1975.

181. Guisasola JA, Cockburn CG, Hardisty RM: Plasma digestion of factor VIII; characterization of the breakdown products with respect to antigenicity and Von Willebrand activity. Thromb Haemostas (Stuttg) 40,302-315,1978.

182. Haakenstad AD, Mannik M: Saturation of the reticulo-endothelial system with soluble immune complexes. J Immunol 112, 1939-1948, 1974.

183. Haljamäe H: Anatomy of the interstitial tissue. Lymphology 11, 128-132, 1978.

184. Hall CL, Hardwicke J: Low molecular weight proteinuria. Ann Rev Med 30, 199-211, 1979.

185. Hansen NE, Karle H, Andersen V: Lysozyme turnover in the rat. J Clin Invest 50, 1473-1477, 1971.

186. Hansen NE, Karle H, Andersen V, Ølgaard K: Lysozyme turnover in man. J Clin Invest 51, 1146-1155, 1972.

187. Hansson HE: Right duct lymph during and after open heart surgery. Scand J Thoracic Cardiovasc Surg 9, 229-239, 1975.

188. Haralambi G, Berg A: Creatine kinase and hexose phosphate isomerase activity in skeletal muscle of healthy male adults. Enzyme 23, 104-107, 1978.

189. Hardonk MJ, Meskendorp-Haarsma TJ, Koudstaal J: A histochemical study about the influence of lytic enzymes on plasma membrane enzyme activities in rat liver and kidney. Histochem 58, 177-181, 1978.

190. Harnarayan C, Bennett MA, Pentecost BL, Brewer DB: Quantitative study of infarcted myocardium in cardiogenic shock. Br Heart J 32, 728-732, 1970.
191. Hasselback R, Hjort PF: Effect of heparin on in vivo turnover of clotting factors. J Appl Physiol 15, 945-948, 1960.
192. Hearse DJ, Humphrey SM, Chain EB: Abrupt reoxygenation of the anoxic potassium - arrested perfused rat heart; a study of myocardial enzyme release. J Mol Cell Cardiol 5, 395-407, 1973.
193. Hearse DJ, Humphrey SM, Garlick PB: Species variation in myocardial anoxic enzyme release, glucose protection and reoxygenation damage. J Mol Cell Cardiol 8, 329-339, 1976.
194. Hearse DJ, Opie LH, Katzeff JE, Lubbe WF, Van der Werff TJ, Peisach M, Boulle G: Characterisation of the "border zone" in acute regional ischemia in the dog. Am J Cardiol 40, 716-725, 1977.
195. Hearse DJ: Cellular damage during myocardial ischemia; metabolic changes leading to enzyme leakage. In: Enzymes in cardiology. DJ Hearse, J de Leiris (eds), John Wiley and Sons,London,1979,1-19.
196. Hearse DJ, Braimbridge MV, Jynge P: Protection of the ischemic myocardium: cardioplegia. New York, Raven Press Books Ltd, 1981.
197. Hearse DJ, Yellon DM: The "border zone" in evolving myocardial infarction; controversy or confusion ? Am J Cardiol 47,1321-1334,1981.
198. Hebert LA, Stuart KA, Allhiser C, Rodey GE: Measurement of the fractional uptake of macromolecules by the renal vascular bed compared to other vascular beds. J Lab Clin Med 87, 716-724, 1976.
199. Hellemans J, Vorlat M, Verstraete M: Survival time of prothrombin and factors VII, IX and X after completely synthesis blocking doses of coumarin derivatives. Br J Haematol 9, 506-512, 1963.
200. Henley KS, Schmidt E, Schmidt FW: Serum enzymes. Clin Sci 174, 119-123, 1960.
201. Henning RJ, Weil MH: Effect of afterload reduction on plasma volume during acute heart failure. Am J Cardiol 42, 823-827, 1978.
202. Hermens WT, Witteveen SAGJ, Hollaar L, Hemker HC: Effect of a thrombolytic agent (urokinase) on necrosis after acute myocardial infarction. In: Recent advances in studies on cardiac structure and metabolism. PE Roy, G Rona (eds), Baltimore, Univ Park Press,1975,vol 10,319-329.
203. Hermens WT, Van der Laarse A, Witteveen SAGJ: Enzymatic infarct sizing; factors influencing the choice of the marker enzyme. In: Enzymes in cardiology. DJ Hearse, J de Leiris (Eds), New York, John Wiley & sons, 1979, 339-353.
204. Herschberg PI, Wells RE, McGandy RB: Hematocrit and prognosis in patients with acute myocardial infarction. JAMA 219, 855-860, 1972.
205. Higuchi M, Nishi K, Takenaka F: A comparison of enzyme activity for energy production in the myocardium and conduction system. Jap Heart J 20, 667-673, 1979.
206. Hirzel HO, Sonnenblick EH, Kirk ES: Absence of a lateral border zone of intermediate creatine phosphokinase depletion surrounding a central infarct 24 hours after acute coronary occlusion in the dog. Circ Res 41, 673-683, 1977.
207. Hitzig WH, Zollinger W: Kongenitaler Faktor-VII-Mangel. Familienuntersuchung und physiologische Studien über den Faktor VII. Helvet Paediat Acta 13, 189-203, 1958.
208. Hjort PF, Egeberg O, Mikkelsen S: Turnover of prothrombin, factor VII and factor IX in a patient with hemophilia A. Scand J Clin Lab Invest 13: 668-672, 1961.
209. Hoag MS, Aggeler PM, Fowell AH: Disappearance rate of concentrated proconvertin extracts in congenital and acquired hypoproconvertinemia. J Clin Invest 39, 554-563, 1960.

210. Hoag MS, Johnson FF, Robinson JA, Aggeler PM: Treatment of hemophilia B with a new clotting - factor concentrate. New Eng J Med 280, 581-586, 1969.

211. Høedt-Rasmussen K, Hasch E, Jarum S: Extravascular degradation of albumin in humans. In: Labelled proteins in tracer studies. L Donato, G Milhaud, J Sirchis (Eds). Brussels, Euratom, 1966, 151-158.

212. Hoffman GC, Hewlett JS: Exchange transfusion in hereditary factor VII (proconvertin) deficiency. Am J Clin Path 44, 198-202, 1965.

213. Hollaar L, Van der Laarse A: Interference of the measurement of lactate dehydrogenase (LDH) activity in human serum and plasma by LDH from blood cells. Clin Chim Acta 99, 135-142, 1979.

214. Horowitz HJ, Fujimoto MM: Survival of factor XI in vitro and in vivo. Transfusion 5, 539-542, 1965.

215. Hossner KL, Billiar RB: Plasma clearance and organ distribution of native and desialylated rat and human transcortin. Species specificity. Endocrinology 108, 1780-1786, 1981.

216. Hovi T, Mosher D, Vaheri A: Cultured human monocytes synthesize and secrete alpha 2-macroglobulin. J Expltl Med 145, 1580-1589, 1977.

217. Hudgson P, Field EJ: Regeneration of muscle. In: The structure and function of muscle. GH Bourne (ED), New York, Acad Press, 1973, vol III, 311-363.

218. Hüttner J, Rona G, More RH: Fibrin deposition within cardiac muscle cells in malignant hypertension. An electron microscopic study. Arch Pathol 91, 19-28, 1971.

219. Ingram GJC, Pinniger JL, Vallet L: Survival in an afibrinogenaemic subject of fibrinogen prepared from "time-expired" blood. Lancet Jan 16, 135-137, 1960.

220. Ingram GJC: Calculating the dose of factor VIII in the management of haemophilia. Br J Haematol 48, 351-354, 1981.

221. Ingwall JS, DeLuca M, Sybers HD, Wildenthal K: Fetal mouse hearts, a model for studying ischemia. Proc Nat Acad Sci USA 72, 2809-2813, 1975.

222. Inoue J, Meda T, Kobatake Y: Structure of exitable membranes formed on the surface of protoplasmic drops isolated from Nitella. Biochim Biophys Acta (biomembranes) 298, 653-663, 1973.

223. Inoue M, Hori M, Nishimoto Y, Fukui S, Abe H, Wada H, Minamino T: Immunological determination of serum m-AST activity in patients with acute myocardial infarction. Br Heart J 40, 1251-1256, 1978.

224. Iio A, Waldmann TA, Strober W: Metabolic study of human IGE: evidence for an extravascular catabolic pathway. J Immunol 120, 1696-1701, 1978.

225. Iseri LT? Balatony EL, Evans JR? Crane MG: Pathogenesis of congestive heart failure. Effect of posture and exercise on plasma volume and plasma constituents. Ann Intern Med 55, 384-394, 1961.

226. Jackson CM, Nemerson Y: Blood coagulation. Ann Rev Biochem 49, 765-811, 1980.

227. Jaenike JR, Schreiner F, Waterhouse C: The relative volumes of distribution of I-131-tagged albumin and high molecular weight dextran in normal subjects and patients with heart disease. J Lab Clin Med, 49, 172-181, 1957.

228. Jaffe EA, Nachman RL: Subunit structure of factor VIII synthesized by cultured human endothelial cells. J Clin Invest 56, 698-702, 1975.

229. Janse MJ, Cinca J, Moréna H, Fiolet JWT, Kléber AG, de Vries GP, Becker AE, Durrer D: The "border zone" in myocardial ischemia. An electrophysiological, metabolic and histochemical correlation in the pig heart. Circ Res 44, 576-588, 1979.

230. Jacquez JA: Compartmental analysis in biology and medicine. Elsevier, Amsterdam, 1972.

231. Jarnum S, Lassen NA: Albumin and transferrin metabolism in infections and toxic diseases. Scand J Clin Lab Invest 13, 357-368, 1961.

232. Jedeikin LA: Regional distribution of glycogen and phosphorylase in the ventricles of the heart. Circ Res 14, 202-211, 1964.

233. Jennings RB, Kaltenbach JP, Smetters GW: Enzymatic changes in acute myocardial ischemic injury. Arch Pathol 64, 10-16, 1957.

234. Jennings RB, Hawkins HK, Lowe JE, Hill ML, Klotman S, Reimer KA: Relation between high energy phosphate and lethal injury in myocardial ischemia in the dog. Am J Pathol 92, 187-215, 1978.

235. Jensen H, Bro-Jørgensen K, Jarnum S, Olesen H, Yssing M: Transferrin metabolism in the nephrotic syndrome and in protein-losing gastroenteropathy. Scand J Clin Lab Invest 21, 293-304, 1968.

236. Jensen KB: Metabolism of human gamma-macroglobulin (IgM) in normal man. Scand J Clin Lab Invest 24, 205-214, 1969.

237. Jewell WR, Krishnan C, Schloerb PR: Apparent cellular ingress of albumin in Walker 256 tumor and rat muscle. Cancer Res 35, 405-408, 1975.

238. Johansson BR: Movement of interstitially microinjected 125-I-labelled albumin into blood capillaries of rat skeletal muscle demonstrated with electron microscopic autoradiography. Microvasc Res 16, 354-361, 1978.

239. Johnson RN, Sammel NL, Norris RM: Depletion of myocardial creatine kinase, lactate dehydrogenase, myoglobin and K+ after coronary artery ligation in dogs. Cardiovasc Res 15,529-537,1981.

240. Johnstone RE, Kennell EN, Brummund W, Shaw LM, Ebersole RC: Effect of halothane anesthesia on muscle, liver, thyroid and adrenal-function tests in man. Clin Chem 22,217-222, 1976.

241. Jones EA, Vergalla J, Steer CJ, Bradley-Moore PR, Vierling JM: Metabolism of intact and desialylated alpha 1-antitrypsin. Clin Sci Mol Med 55, 139-148, 1978.

242. Jones P, Martin-Villar J, De Vreker R, Taub R: Management of the hemophilias. Scand J Haematol 24, suppl 35, 1980.

243. Josso F, Prou-Wartelle O, Charlas J: Durée de vie du facteur Hageman (facteur XII). Nouv Rev Fr Hematol 4, 454-456, 1964.

244. Kahn JC, Gueret P, Menier R, Giraudet P, Ben Farhat M, Bourdarias JP: Prognostic value of enzymatic (CPK) estimation of infarct size. J Mol Med 2, 223-231, 1977.

245. Kane JP: Plasma lipoproteins: structure and metabolism. In: Lipid metabolism in mammals. F Snyder (Ed), New York, Plenum Press, 1977, vol I, 209-257.

246. Karmen A: A note on the spectrophotometric assay of glutamic-oxaloacetic transaminase in human blood serum. J Clin Invest 34, 131-133, 1955.

247. Katz JH: Iron and protein kinetics studied by means of doubly labeled human crystalline transferrin. J Clin Invest 40, 2143-2152, 1961.

248. Katz J, Bonorris G, Golden S, Sellers AL: Extravascular albumin mass and exchange in rat tissues. Clin Sci 39, 705-724, 1970.

249. Katz J, Bonorris G, Sellers AL: Extravascular albumin in human tissues. Clin Sci 39, 725-729, 1970.

250. Kay HD: Plasma phosphatase in osteitis deformans and in other diseases of bone. Br J Exp Path 10, 253-256, 1929.

251. Kedem O, Essig A: Isotope flows and flux ratios in biological membranes. J Gen Physiol 48, 1047-1070, 1965.

253. Kent SP: Diffusion of plasma proteins into cells; a manifestation of cell injury in human myocardial ischemia. Am J Pathol 50, 623-637, 1967.

254. Kernoff LM, Baker G: Direct measurement of transferrin synthesis rates in man using the 14C carbonate method. Anal Biochem 106, 529-534, 1980.

255. Kibe O, Nilsson NJ: Observations on the diagnostic and prognostic value of some enzyme tests in myocardial infarction. Acta Med Scand 182, 597-

610, 1967.

256. Kirk ES, Honig CR: Nonuniform distribution of blood flow and gradients of oxygen tension within the heart. Am J Physiol 207, 661-668, 1964.

257. Kjekshus JK, Sobel BE: Depressed myocardial creatine phosphokinase activity following experimental myocardial infarction in rabbit. Circ Res 27, 403-414, 1970.

258. Kloner RA, Braunwald E: Observations on experimental myocardial ischemia. Cardiovasc Res 14, 371-395, 1980.

259. Kluthe R, Hagemann U, Kleine N: The turnover of alpha 2-macroglobulins in the nephrotic syndrome. Vox Sang 12, 308-311, 1967.

260. Kobayashi N, Takeda Y: Effects of a large dose of oestradiol on antithrombin III metabolism in male and female dogs. Eur J Clin Invest 7, 373-381, 1977.

261. Kohler PF, Müller-Eberhard HJ: Metabolism of human C1q. Studies in hypogammaglobulinemia, myeloma and systemic lupus erythematosus. J Clin Invest 51, 868-875, 1972.

262. Koj A: Acute-phase reactants. Their synthesis, turnover and biological significance. In: Structure and function of plasma proteins, vol 1; AC Allison (Ed), Plenum Press, London, 1974, 73-131.

263. Koskelo P, Kekki M, Nikkilä EA, Virkkunen M: Turnover of 131-I-labelled ceruloplasmin in rheumatoid arthritis. Scand J Clin Lab Invest 19, 259-262, 1967.

264. Koskelo P, Kekki M, Mustajoki P, Valmet E: Turnover of 125-I-labeled hemopexin in man. Enzyme 17, 116-121, 1974.

265. Kouchonkos NT, Oberman A, Kirklin JW: Coronary bypass surgery; analysis of factors effecting hospital mortality. Circulation 62, Suppl 1, 184-189,1980.

266. Kung-Ming J, Chien S, Bigger J: Observations on blood viscosity changes after acute myocardial infarction. Circulation, 51, 1079-1084, 1975.

267. Kushner I, Feldmann G: Control of the acute phase response. Demonstration of C-Reactive protein synthesis and secretion by hepatocytes during acute inflammation in the rabbit. J Exp Med 148, 466-477, 1978.

268. Kushner I, Broder MI, Karp D: Control of the acute phase response. Serum C-reactive protein kinetics after acute myocardial infarction. J Clin Invest 61, 235-242, 1978.

269. LaDue JS, Wróblewski F, Karmen A: Serum glutamic oxaloacetic transaminase activity in human acute transmural myocardial infarction. Science 120, 497-499, 1954.

270. Lal-Choudhury S, Edge JR, Stansfield D: Serum fibrin/fibrinogen degradation products as a prognostic index in acute myocardial infarction. J Clin Path 28, 821-824, 1975.

271. Lamerz R, Fateh-Moghadam A: Übersichten. Carcinofetale Antigene. I. Alpha-Fetoprotein. Klin Wschr 53, 147-169, 1975.

272. Lane RS, Rangeley DM, Liem HH, Wormsley S, Müller-Eberhard U: Hemopexin metabolism in the rabbit. J Lab Clin Med 79, 935-941, 1972.

273. Langer T, Strober W, Levy RJ: The metabolism of low density lipoprotein in familial type II hyperlipoproteinemia. J Clin Invest 51, 1528-1536, 1972.

274. Lassen NA, Parving HH, Rossing N: Filtration as the main mechanism of overall transcapillary protein escape from the plasma. Microvasc Res 7, i-iv, 1974.

275. Laurell CB, Nosslin B, Jeppsson JO: Catabolic rate of alpha 1-antitrypsin of Pi type M and Z in man. Clin Sci Mol Med 52, 457-461, 1977.

276. Lavergne JM, Josso F: Metabolism of Pivaka in man. In: Prothrombin and related coagulation factors. Boerhaave series for postgraduate medical education nr. 10, HC Hemker, JJ Veltkamp (Eds), Leiden, Univ Press, 1975,

167-190.

277. Lewallen CG, Berman M, Rall JE: Studies of iodo-albumin metabolism I. A mathematical approach to the kinetics. J Clin Invest 38, 66-87, 1959.

278. Lewallen CG, Rall JE, Berman M: Studies of Iodo-albumin metabolism II. Effects of thyroid hormone. J Clin Invest 38, 88-101, 1959.

279. Lewis JH, Ferguson EE, Schoenfeld C: Studies concerning the turnover of fibrinogen I-131 in the dog. J Lab Clin Med 58, 247-258, 1961.

280. Liem HH: Catabolism of homologous and heterologous hemopexin in the rat and uptake of hemopexin by isolated perfused rat liver. Ann Clin Res 8, Suppl 17, 233-238, 1976.

281. Loeliger EA, Van der Esch B, Mattern MJ, Hemker HC: The Biological disappearance rate of prothrombin, factors VII, IX and X from plasma in hypothyroidism, hyperthyroidism and during fever. Thrombos Diathes Haemorrh 10, 267-277, 1964.

282. Loeliger EA, Hensen A, Mattern MJ, Veltkamp JJ, Bruning PF, Hemker HC: Treatment of haemophilia B with purified factor IX (PPSB): Folia Med Neerl 10, 112-125, 1967.

283. Löhr GW, Waller HD: Zellstoffwechsel und Zellalterung. Klin Wschr 37, 833-843, 1959.

284. Losowsky MS, Leeds MD, Hall R, Goldie W: Congenital deficiency of fibrin-stabilising factor. Lancet, Vol II (july 24), 156-158, 1965.

285. Lumry R, Biltonen R, Brandts JF: Validity of the "twostate" hypothesis for conformational transitions of proteins. Biopolymers 4, 917-944, 1966.

286. Lundsgaard-Hansen P, Meyer C, Riedwyl H: Transmural gradients of glycolytic enzyme activity in left ventricular myocardium. Pflügers Archiv 297, 89-106, 1967.

287. Macchia DD, Page E, Polimeni PI: Interstitial anion distribution in striated muscle determined with 35-S sulfate and 3-H sucrose. Am J Physiol 237, C125-C130, 1979.

288. McFarlane AS: Efficient trace-labelling of proteins with Iodine. Nature 183, 53, 1958.

289. McFarlane AS: In vivo behavior of I-131-fibrinogen. J Clin Invest 42, 346-361, 1963.

290. McFarlane AS: Measurement of synthesis rates of liver-produced proteins. Biochem J 89, 277-290, 1963.

291. McFarlane AS, Todd D, Cromwell S: Fibrinogen catabolism in humans. Clin Sci 26, 415-420, 1964.

292. McFarlane AS, Koj A: Short-term measurement of catabolic rates using iodine-labeled plasma proteins. J Clin Invest 49, 1903-1911, 1970.

293. McMillan CW, Webster WP, Roberts HR, Blythe WB: Continuous intravenous infusion of factor VIII in classic haemophilia. Br J Haematol 18, 659-667, 1970.

294. Mahey BWJ, Rowson KEK, Parr CW, Salaman MH: Studies on the mechanism of action of Riley virus. I. Action of substances affecting the reticuloendothelial system on plasma enzyme levels in mice. J Exptl Med 122, 967-981, 1965.

295. Mahey BWJ, Rowson KEK, Parr CW: Studies on the mechanism of action of Riley virus IV. The reticuloendothelial system and impaired plasma enzyme clearance in infected mice. J Exptl Med 125, 277-288, 1967.

296. Makino S, Reed CE: Distribution and elimination of exogenous alpha$_1$-antitrypsin. J Lab Clin Med 75, 742-746, 1970.

297. Malmberg P: Enzyme composition of dog heart lymph after myocardial infarction. Upsala J Med Sci 78, 73-77, 1973.

298. Marland M, Hansman, FS, Robison R: The phosphoric-esterase of blood. Biochem J 18, 1152-1160, 1924.

299. Maroko PR, Maclean D, Ribeiro LGT, Braunwald E: Pharmacolocgial limita-

tion of infarct size: enzymatic, electrocardiographic and morphological studies in the experimental animal and man. In: Enzymes in cardiology. J Hearse, J De Leiris (Eds), New York, John Wiley and Sons, 1979, 529-559.

300. Massarrat S: Verhalten und Schwundrate der Glutamat-Oxalacetat- Transaminase in der Blutbahn. Z Ges Exp Med 148, 56-71, 1968.

301. Matthews CME: The theory of tracer experiments with 131-I labeled plasma proteins. Physics Med Biol 2, 36-53, 1957.

302. Meyer K, Eernisse JG, Veltkamp JJ, Hemker HC, Loeliger EA: Treatment of haemophilia A with purified factor VIII obtained from human plasma by cryoprecipitation. Folia Med Neerl 10, 49-60, 1967.

303. Mezger VA, Kahles H, Stellwaag M, Spieckermann PG: Myoglobin and enzymes: simultaneously liberated diagnostic markers of myocardial cell damage. J Mol Cell Cardiol 11, 37, 1979.

304. Miescher PA: Circulating complement breakdown products in patients with rheumatoid arthritis. Correlation between plasma C3d, circulating immune complexes and clinical activity. J Clin Invest 59, 862-868, 1977.

305. Miller LL, Hanavan HR, Titthasiri N, Chowdhury A: Dominant role of the liver in biosynthesis of plasma proteins with special reference to the plasma mucoproteins (seromucoid), ceruloplasmin and fibrinogen. Adv Chem Ser 44, 17-40, 1964.

306. Miloszewski K, Losowsky MS: The half-life of factor XIII in vivo. Br J Haematol 19, 685-690, 1970.

307. Mohiuddin SM, Raffetto J, Sketch MH, Lynch JD, Schultz RD, Runco V: LDH isoenzymes and myocardial infarction in patients undergoing coronary bypass surgery: an excellent correlation. Am Heart J 92, 584-588, 1976.

308. Molander DW, Wroblewsky F, La Due JS: Serum glutamic oxalacetic transaminase as an index of hepatocellular integrity. J Lab Clin Med 46,831-839,1955.

309. Morell A, Terry WD, Waldmann TA: Metabolic properties of IgG subclases in man. J Clin Invest 49, 673-680, 1970.

310. Morell A, Skvaril F, Noseda G, Barandun S: Metabolic properties of human IgA subclasses. Clin Exp Immunol 13, 521-528, 1973.

311. Morin LG: Creatine kinase isoenzyme-antibody reactions in immuno inhibition and immuno-nephelometry.Clin Chem 25, 1415-1419, 1979.

312. Mouridsen HT: Turnover of human serum albumin before and after operations. Clin Sci 33, 345-354, 1967.

313. Myant NB: Observations om the metabolism of human gamma-globulin labeled by radioactive iodine. Clin Sci 11,191-201,1952.

314. Nakai T, Whayne TF: Catabolism of canine apolipoprotein A-1: Purification catabolic rate, organs of catabolism and the liver subcellular catabolic site. J Lab Clin Med 88, 63-80, 1976.

315. Nayler WG, Slade AM: Pharmacological protection of the hypoxic heart: enzymatic, biochemical and ultrastructural studies in the isolated heart. In: Enzymes in cardiology. DJ Hearse, J de Leiris (Eds), New York, John Wiley and sons, 1979, 503-521.

316. Nealon DA, Henderson AR: Creatine kinase-1 is prinicpally inactivated in serum by complexing with immunoglobulin G. Clin Sci 58, 157-160, 1980.

317. Neil WA, Levine HJ, Wagman RJ, Messer JV, Krasnow N, Gorlin R: Ventricular heat production measured by coronary flow and temperature gradient. J Appl Physiol 16, 883-890, 1961.

318. Nenci GG, Agnelli G, De Regis FM: Coag kinetics on factor-VII-CRM[+] and factor-VII-CRM[-] deficiencies. Br J Haematol 46, 307-309, 1980.

319. Neutze JM, Drakeley MJ, Barratt-Boyes BG, Hubbert K: Serum enzymes after cardiac surgery using cardiopulmonary bypass. Am Heart J 88, 425-442, 1974.

320. Nicolaysen G: Protein concentration in lymph. Lymphology 11, 143-146,

1978.

321. Neuhaus OW, Balegno HF, Chandler AM: Induction of plasma protein synthesis in response to trauma. Am J Physiol, 211, 151-156, 1966.

322. Nieuwenhuizen W, Emeis JF, Vermond A, Kurver P, Van der Heide D: Studies on the catabolism and distribution of fibrinogen in rats. Application of the iodogen R labelling technique. Biochem Biophys Res Commun 97, 49-55, 1980.

323. Niléhn J-E, Ganrot PO: Plasmin, plasmin inhibitors and degradation products of fibrinogen in human serum during and after intravenous infusion of streptokinase. Scand J Clin Lab Invest 20, 113-121, 1967.

324. Nilsson-Ehle P: Lipolytic enzymes and plasma lipoprotein metabolism. Ann Rev Biochem 49, 667-693, 1980.

325. Nisimoto S: Study on transaminiase. Kyushu J Med Sci 8, 139-154, 1957.

326. Nora JJ, Cooley DA, Fernbach DJ, Rochelle DG, Milham JD, Montgomery JR, Leachman RD, Butler WT, Rossen RD, Bloodwell RD, Hallman GL, Trenton JJ: Rejection of the transplanted human heart. Indexes of recognition and problems in prevention. New Eng J Med 280, 1079-1086, 1969.

327. Nordbeck H, Kahles H, Preusse CJ, Spieckermann PG: Enzymes in cardiac lymph and coronary blood under normal and pathophysiological conditions. J Mol Med 2, 255-263, 1977.

328. Norris RM, Whitlock RML, Barratt-Boyes C, Small CW:Clinical measurement of myocardial infarct size. Modification of a method for the estimation of total creatine phosphokinase release after myocardial infarction. Circulation 51, 614-620, 1975.

329. Norris RM, Howell D, Whitlock RLM, Heng MK, Peter T: Enzyme release after myocardial infarction; comparison of serial serum alpha-hydroxybutyrate dehydrogenase with creatine kinase levels. Eur J Cardiol 4, 461-468, 1976.

330. Nossel HL, Niemetz J, Sawitsky A: Blood PTA (factor XI) levels following plasma infusion. Proc Soc Exp Biol Med 115, 896-900, 1964.

331. Nosslin B: Nosslin's modification of the model C of Reeve and Roberts. In: Andersen SB: Metabolism of human gamma globulin. Blackwell Publ, Oxford 1964.

332. Nosslin B: Analysis of disappearance time-curves after single injection of labelled proteins. In: Protein turnover. Ciba Found Symp 9 (new series). Amsterdam, Elsevier, 1973, 113-130.

333. Noyes WD, Garby L: Rate of haptoglobin in synthesis in normal man. Determinations by the return to normal levels following hemoglobin infusion. Scand J Clin Lab Invest 20, 33-38, 1967.

334. Nydick J, Wróblewski F, LaDue JS: Evidence for increased serum glutamic oxalacetic transaminase (SGOT) activity following graded myocardial infarcts in dogs. Circulation 12, 161-168, 1955.

335. Oldham HN, Roe CR, Young WG, Dixon SH: Intraoperative detection of myocardial damage during coronary artery surgery by plasma creatine phosphokinase isoenzyme analysis. Surgery 74, 917-925, 1973.

336. Olesen H: Turnover studies with iodine-labeled gamma-macroglobulin and albumin. Scand J Clin Lab Invest 15, 497-510, 1963.

337. Olszewski WL, Loe K, Engeset A: Immune proteins and other biochemical constituents of peripheral lymph in patients with malignancy and post-irraÙiation lymphedema. Lymphology 11, 174-180, 1978.

338. Oppenheimer JH, Surks MJ, Bernstein G, Smith JC: Metabolism of Iodine-131-labeled thyroxine-binding prealbumin in man. Science 149, 748-750, 1965.

339. Oratz M: Oncotic pressure and albumin synthesis. In: Plasma protein metabolism. MA Rothschild, T Waldmann (eds), Acad Press, New York, 1970, 223-238.

340. Orrenius S, Thor H, Rajs J, Berggren M: Isolated rate hepatocytes as an experimental tool in the study of cell injury. Effect of anoxia. Forensic Science 8, 255-263, 1976.

341. Over J, Sixma JJ, Doucet-de Bruïne MHM, Trieschnigg AMC, Vlooswijk RAA, Beeser-Visser NH, Bouma BN: Survival of 125 Iodine-labeled factor VIII in normals and patients with classic hemophilia. Observations on the heterogeneity of human factor VIII. J Clin Invest 62: 223-234, 1978.

342. Over J, Sixma JJ, Bouma BN, Bolhuis PA, Vlooswijk RAA, Beeser-Visser NH: Survival of iodine-125-labeled factor VIII in patients with von Willebrand's disease. J Lab Clin Med 97, 332-344, 1981.

343. Owen CA, Mann KG, McDuffie FC: The turnover in normal dogs of prothrombin and its fragments; effect of induced intravascular coagulation. Thrombos Haemostas (Stuttg) 42, 548-555, 1979.

344. Packard CJ, Third JLHC, Shepherd J, Lorimer AR, Morgan HG, Lawrie TDV: Low density lipoprotein metabolism in a family of familial hypercholesterolemic patients. Metabolism 25, 995-1006, 1976.

345. Page DL, Caulfield JB, Kastor JA, De Sanctis RW, Sanders CA: Myocardial changes associated with cardiogenic shock. New Eng J Med 285, 133-137, 1971.

346. Pappenheimer JR: Passage of molecules through capillary walls. Physiol Rev 33, 387-423, 1953.

347. Parving H-H, Gyntelberg F: Transcapillary escape rate of albumin and plasma volume in essential hypertension. Circ Res 32, 643-651, 1973.

348. Parving H-H, Jensen HAE, Westrup M: Increased transcapillary escape rate of albumin and IgG in essential hypertension. Scand J Clin Lab Invest 37, 223-227, 1977.

349. Peppard JV, Orlans E: The biological half-lives of four rat immunoglobulin isotypes. Immunology 40, 683-686, 1980.

350. Peterson PA, Nilsson SF, Ostberg L, Rask L, Vahlquist A: Aspects of the metabolism of retinol-binding protein and retinol. Vit Horm 32, 181-214, 1974.

351. Petersen VP, Ottosen P: Albumin turnover and thoracic-duct lymph in constrictive pericarditis. Acta Med Scand 176, 335-344, 1964.

352. Petz LD, Fink DJ, Letsky EA, Fudenberg HH, Müller-Eberhard HJ: In vivo metabolism of complement I. Metabolism of the third component (C3) in acquired hemolytic anemia. J Clin Invest 47, 2469-2484, 1968.

353. Pflughaupt KW: Cerebrogenic enzymes. In: Advances in clinical enzymology. E Schmidt, FW schmidt, J Trautschold, R Friedel (Eds). Basel, S Karger, 1979, 136-142.

354. Pool JG, Welton J, Creger WP: Ineffectiveness of intramuscularly injected factor VIII concentrate in two hemophilic patients. New Eng J Med 275, 547-548, 1966.

355. Porter RR: The croonian lecture 1980; the complex proteases of the complement system. Proc R Soc London B 210, 477-498, 1980.

356. Posen S: Turnover of circulating enzymes. Clin Chem 16, 71-84, 1970.

357. Putnam FW: The plasma proteins structure, function and genetic control. Vol 1, Academic Press, New York, 1975, 2nd ed.

358. Qureshi AR, Wilkinson JH: The fate of circulating lactate dehydrogenase-5 in the rabbit. Clin Sci Mol Med 50, 1-14, 1976.

359. Rapaport E: The fractional disappearance rate of the separate isoenzymes of creatine phosphokinase in the dog. Cardiovasc Res 9, 473-477, 1975.

360. Ravens KG, Gubbjarnason S, Cowan CM, Bing RJ: Gamma-glutamyl-transpeptidase in myocardial infarction. Clinical and experimental studies. Circulation XXXIX, 693-700, 1969.

361. Reeve EB, Roberts JE: The catabolism of plasma albumin in the rabbit. Its rate and regulation. J Gen Physiol 43, 445-453, 1959.

362. Reeve EB, Bailey HR: Mathematical models describing the distribution of I-131-albumin in man. J Lab Clin Med 60, 923-943, 1962.
363. Reeve EB, Pearson JR, Martz DC: Plasma protein synthesis in the liver. Method for measurement of albumin formation in vivo. Science 139, 914-916, 1963.
365. Reeve EB, Chen Y: Studies with a mass balance method of measuring fibrinogen synthesis. In: Protein turnover. Ciba Foundation Symposium 9 (new series) Elsevier Exerpta Medica North-Holland, 1973, 91-112.
366. Refetoff S, Fang VS, Marshall JS, Robin NJ: Metabolism of thyroxine-binding globulin in man. Abnormal rate of synthesis in inherited thyroxine-binding globulin deficiency and excess. J Clin Invest 57, 485-495, 1976.
367. Regoeczi E, Regoeczi GE, McFarlane AS: Relation between rate of catabolism, plasma concentration and pool size of fibrinogen. Pflügers Arch Ges Physiol 279, 17-25, 1964.
368. Regoeczi E: Fibrinogen catabolism: kinetics of catabolism following sudden elevation of the pool with exogenous fibrinogen. Clin Sci 38, 111-121, 1970.
369. Regoeczi E, Koj A, Lam LSL: Synthesis and catabolism of rabbit alpha 1-antitrypsins F and S. Biochem J 192, 929-934, 1980.
370. Reichard H: Ornithine carbamyl transferase in dog serum on intravenous injection of enzyme, choledochus ligation and carbon tetrachloride poisoning. J Lab Clin Med 53, 417-425, 1959.
371. Renkin EM: Multiple pathways of capillary permeability. Circ Res 41, 735-743, 1977.
372. Renkin EM, Curry FE: Transport of water and solutes across capillary endothelium. In: Membrane transport in biology. G Giebisch, DC Tosteson, HH Ussing (Eds), Berlin, Springer Verlag, 1979, vol IV A, 1-45.
373. Rennie JAN, Ogston D: Changes in coagulation factors following acute myocardial infarction in man. Haemostasis 5, 258-264, 1976.
374. Rescigno A: A contribution to the theory of tracer methods II. Biochim Biophys Acta 21, 111-116, 1956.
375. Reuge C, Blatrix C, Brevet JP, Steinbruch M: Etude de la demie-vie de l' alpha 2-macroglobuline. In: Labelled proteins in tracer studies. L Donato, G Milhaud, J Sirchis (Eds) Brussels, Euratom 1966, 143-149.
376. Revis NW, Thomson RY, Cameron AJV: Lactate dehydrogenase isoenzymes in the human hypertrophic heart. Cardiovasc Res 11, 172-176, 1977.
377. Revis NW, Cameron AJV: Association of myocardial cell necrosis with experimental cardiac hypertrophy. J Pathol 128, 193-202, 1979.
378. Rippe B, Lundin S, Folkow B: Plasma volume, blood volume and transcapillary escape rate of albumin in young spontaneously hypertensive rats as compared with normotensive controls. Clin Exp Hypertension 1, 39-50, 1978.
379. Rippe B, Kamiya A, Folkow B: Transcapillary passage of albumin, effects of tissue cooling and of increases in filtration and plasma colloid osmotic pressure. Acta Physiol Scand 105, 171-187, 1979.
380. Roberts HR, Lechler E, Webster WP, Peninck GD: Survival of transfused factor X in patients with stuart disease. Thromb Diath Haemorrh 13, 305-313, 1965.
381. Roberts R, Henry PD, Sobel BE: An improved basis for enzymatic estimation of infarct size. Circulation 52, 743-754, 1975.
382. Roberts R, Sobel BE: Effect of selected drugs and myocardial infarction on the disappearance of creatine kinase from the circulation in conscious dogs. Cardiovasc Res 11, 103-112, 1977.
383. Robison AK, Gnepp DR, Sobel BE: Inactivation of CPK in lymph. Circulation 52, Suppl II, 5, 1975.
384. Roe CR, Starmer CF: A sensitivity analysis of enzymatic estimation of

infarct size. Circulation 52, 1-5, 1975.

385. Roe CR, Frederick RC, Starmer CF: The relationship between enzymatic and histologic estimates of the extent of myocardial infarction in conscious dogs with permanent coronary occlusion. Circulation 55, 438-449, 1977.

386. Roe CR, Wagner GS, Young WG, Curtis SE, Cobb FR, Irvin RG: Relation of creatine kinase isoenzyme MB to postoperative electrocardiographic diagnosis in patients undergoing coronary-artery bypass surgery. Clin Chem 25, 93-98, 1979.

387. Rogentine GN, Rowe DS, Bradley J, Waldmann TA, Fahey JL: Metabolism of human immunoglobulin D (IgD). J Clin Invest 45, 1467-1478, 1966.

388. Roheim PS, Rachmilewitz D, Stein O, Stein Y: Metabolism of iodinated high density lipoproteins in the rat I. Half-life in the circulation and uptake by organs. Biochim Biophys Acta 248, 315-329, 1971.

389. Rona G, Boutet M, Huttner I: Membrane permiability alterations as manifestations of early cardiac muscle cell injury. In: Recent advances in studies on cardiac structure and metabolism. A Fleckenstein, G Rona (eds). Baltimore, Univ Park Press, 1975, vol 6, 439-451.

390. Rosalki SB: Serum alpha-hydroxybutyrate dehydrogenase; a new test for myocardial infarction. Br Heart J 25, 795-802, 1963.

391. Rosenoer VM, Oratz M, Rothschild MA: Albumin, structure, function and uses. Pergamon Press Inc, New York, 1977.

392. Rosenthal RL, Sloan E: PTA (factor XI) levels and coagulation studies after plasma infusions in PTA-deficient patients. J Lab Clin Med 66, 709-714, 1965.

393. Rossing N, Jensen H: Metabolic studies of different albumin preparations. Clin Sci 32, 89-99, 1967.

394. Rothschild MA, Oratz M, Schreiber SS: Serum Albumin. Am J Digest Dis (new series) 14, 711-744, 1969.

395. Rothschild MA, Waldmann T: Plasma protein metabolism. New York, Acad Press, 1970.

396. Rothschild MA, Oratz M, Schreiber SS: Extravascular albumin. N Engl J Med 301, 497-498, 1979.

397. Rouvier J, Collen D, Swart ACW, Verstraete M: Prothrombin metabolism in healthy subjects and in two patients with congenital hypoprothrombin and related coagulation factors. HC Hemker, JJ Veltkamp (Eds). Leiden, Univ Press, 1975, 167-190.

398. Ruddy S, Carpenter CB, Chin KW, Knostman JN, Soter NA, Gotze O, Müller-Eberhard HJ, Austen KF: Human complement metabolism - an analysis of 144 studies. Medicine 54, 165-178, 1975.

399. Ruegsegger P, Nydick J, Freiman A, LaDue JS: Serum activity patterns of glutamic oxaloacetic transaminase, glutamic pyruvic transaminase and lactic dehydrogenase following graded myocardial infarction in dogs. Circ Res 7, 4-10, 1959.

400. Rutili G, Arfors KE: Protein concentration in interstitial and lymphatic fluids from the subcutaneous tissue. Acta Physiol Scand 99, 1-8, 1977.

401. Rutili G: Transport of macromolecules in subcutaneous tissue studied by FITC-dextrans. Acta Universitatis Upsaliensis (Abstracts of Upsala dissertations from the faculty of Medicine) 306, 1978.

402. Sabiston BH, Rose JEM: Effect of cold exposure on the metabolism of immunoglobulins in rabbits. J Immunol 116, 106-111, 1976.

403. Sachsenheimer W, Goody RS, Schirmer RH: Elimination und Exkretion von Adenylatkinasen nach Zellschädigungen. Klin Wschr 53, 617-622, 1975.

404. Savitz D, Sidel VW, Solomon AK: Osmotic properties of human red cells. J Gen Physiol 48, 79-94, 1964.

405. Schaefer EJ, Eisenberg S, Levy RJ: Lipoprotein apoprotein metabolism. J Lipid Res 19, 667-687, 1978.

406. Schaper J, Mulch J, Winkler B, Schaper W: Ultrastructural, functional and biochemical criteria for estimation of reversibility of ischemic injury; a study on the effects of global ischemia on the isolated dog heart. J Mol Cell Cardiol 11, 521-541, 1979.

407. Schapira F, Dreyfuss JC, Schapira G: La duree de sejour dans la plasma de l'aldolase chez le lapin; etude a l'aide d'une aldolase marquee a l'iode radioactif. Rev Fr Etudes Clin Biol 7, 829-832, 1962.

408. Schmidt E, Schmidt FW: Enzymmuster menschlicher Gewebe. Klin Wschr 38, 957-962, 1960.

409. Schmidt E, Schmidt FW, Herfarth C, Opitz K, Vogell W: Studien zum Austritt von Zell-Enzymen am Modell der isolierten, perfundierten Rattenleber. Enzym Biol Clin 7, 185-202, 1966.

410. Schmidt E, Schmidt FW, Otto P: Isoenzymes of malic dehydrogenase, glutamic oxaloacetic transaminase and lactate dehydrogenase in serum in diseases of the liver. Clin Chim Acta 15, 283-289, 1967.

411. Schmidt E: Enzym-Austritt. In: Praktische Enzymologie. FW Schmidt, H Huber (Eds), Bern, Hans Huber, 1968, 93-148.

412. Schmidt E, Schmidt FW: Enzyme activities in human liver. Enzym Biol Clin 11, 67-129, 1970.

413. Schmidt E, Schmidt FW: Clinical aspects of gut enzymology. J Clin Chem Clin Biochem 17, 693-704, 1979.

414. Schmidt E, Schmidt FW, Trautschold J, Friedel R: Advances in clinical enzymology. Basel, S Karger, 1979.

415. Schreiber SS, Bauman A, Yalow RS, Berson SA: Blood volume alternations in congestive heart failure. J Clin Invest 33, 578-586, 1954.

416. Schuh FT: Serum cholinesterase, effect on the action of suxamethonium following administration to a patient with cholinesterase deficiency. Br J Anesth 49, 269-272, 1977.

417. Schultze HE, Heremans JF: Molecular biology of human proteins. Amsterdam, Elsevier Publ Cy 1966, vol I.

418. Schur PH: Human gamma-G subclasses. Progr Clin Immunol 1, 71-104, 1972.

419. Sears DA: Depletion of plasma hemopexin in man by hematin injections. Proc Soc Exp Biol Med 131, 371-373, 1969.

420. Sedziwy L, Thomas M, Shillingford J: Some observations on hematocrit changes in patients with acute myocardial infarction. Br Heart J 30, 344-349, 1968.

421. Seeman P: Ultrastructure of membrane lesions in immune lysis, osmotic lysis and drug-induced lysis. Fed Proc 33, 2116-2124, 1974.

422. Sell S: Synthesis, equilibration and catabolism of alpha 1 F during gestation and in hepatoma bearing rats. In: L'alpha foeto-proteine. R. Masseyeff (Ed), Paris, Inserm, 1974.

423. Shapiro SS, Martinez J: Human prothrombin metabolism in normal man and in hypocoagulable subjects. J Clin Invest 48, 1292-1298, 1969.

424. Shell WE, Kjekshus JK, Sobel BE: Quantitative assessment of the extent of myocardial infarction in the conscious dog by means of analysis of serial changes in serum creatine phosphokinase activity. J Clin Invest 50, 2614-2625, 1971.

425. Shell WE, Lavelle JF, Covell JW, Sobel BE: Early estimation of myocardial damage in conscious dogs and patients with evolving acute myocardial infarction. J Clin Invest 52, 2579-2590, 1973.

426. Shepp M, Yamada H, Berenfeld M, Gabuzda TG: 125-I-transferrin turnover in rabbits with haemolytic anaemia. Br J Haematol 24, 261-266, 1973.

427. Shirey EK, Proudfit WL, Sones FM: Serum enzyme and electrocardiographic changes after coronary artery surgery . Correlation with selective cine coronary arteriography and left ventriculography. Chest 57, 122-130, 1970.

428. Sibley JA: Significance of serum aldolase levels. Ann NY Acad Sci 75, 339-348, 1958/1959.
429. Sigurdsson G, Nicoll A, Lewis B: Metabolism of very low denisty lipoproteins in Hyperlipidaemia. Studies of apolipoprotein B kinetics in man. Eur J Clin Invest 6, 167-177, 1976.
430. Sissons JGP, Liebowitch J, Amos N, Peters DK: Metabolism of the fifth component of complement and its relation to metabolism of the third component in patients with complement activation. J Clin Invest 59, 704-715, 1977.
431. Sivertssen E, Semb G, Klaebo G, Smith P, Hol R: Myocardial infarction after aortocoronary bypass surgery. The incidence in 187 consecutive patients and the late postoperative significance. Scand J Thor Cardiovasc Surg 14, 67-76, 1980.
432. Slater EC, Rosing J, Mol A: The phosphorylation potential generated by respiring mitochondria. Biochim Biophys Acta 292, 534-553, 1973.
433. Smallwood RA, Jones EA, Craigie A, Raia S, Rosenoer VM: The delivery of newly synthesized albumin and fibrinogen to the plasma in dogs. Clin Sci 35, 35-43, 1968.
434. Smith AF: Diagnostic value of serum creatine kinase in a coronary care unit. Lancet 2, 178-182, 1967.
435. Smith AF, Wong PC-P, Oliver MF: Release of mitochondrial enzymes in acute myocardial infarction. J Mol Med 2, 265-269, 1977.
436. Smith SJ, Bos G, Hagemeyer F, Hermens WT, Witteveen SAGJ: Influences of changes in plasma volume on quantitation of infarct size in man by means of plasma enzyme levels. J Mol Med 1, 199-210, 1976.
437. Smith SJ, Bos G, Esseveld MR, van Eijk HG, Gerbrandy J: Acute phase proteins from the liver and enzymes from myocardial infarction; a quantitative relationship. Clin Chim Acta 81, 75-85, 1977.
438. Snyder S, Durham BC, Ikandrian AS, Coodley EL, Linhart JW: Serum lipids and glycoproteins in acute myocardial infarction. Am Heart J 90, 582-586, 1975.
439. Sobel BE, Bresnahan GF, Shell WE, Yoder RD: Estimation of infarct size in man and its relation to prognosis. Circulation 46, 640-648, 1972.
440. Sobel BE, Markham J, Karlsberg RP, Roberts R: The nature of disappearance of creatine kinase from the circulation and its influences on enzymatic estimation of infarct size. Circ Res 41, 836-844, 1977.
441. Sodetz JM, Pizzo SV, McKee PA: Relationship of sialic acid to function and in vivo survival of human factor VIII/ von Willebrand factor protein. J Biol Chem 252, 5538-5546, 1977.
442. Solomon A, Waldmann TA, Fahey JL: Metabolism of normal 6.6 S gamma-globulin in normal subjects and in patients with macroglobulinemia and multiple myeoloma. J Lab Clin Med 62, 1-17, 1963.
443. Soltys HD, Brody JZ: Synthesis of transferrin by human peripheral blood lymphocytes. J Lab Clin Med 75, 250-257, 1970.
444. Soulier JP, Prou-Wartelle O, Josso F: Demi-vie de la prothrombine vraie (facteur II). Nouv Rev Fr Hematol 2, 673-684, 1962.
445. Spieckermann PG, Nordbeck H, Preusse CJ: From heart to plasma. In: Enzymes in cardiology. DJ Hearse, J de Leiris (eds), John Wiley and sons, New York, 1979, 81-96.
446. Stables DP, Rubenstein AH, Metz J, Levin NW: The possible role of hemoconcentration in the etiology of myocardial infarction. Am Heart J 73, 155-159, 1967.
447. Stähelin HB: 75 Se-Selenomethionine-labeled lipoproteins in hyperlipidemic and normolipidemic humans. Metabolism 24, 505-515, 1975.
448. Steele P, Rainwater J: Relationship of plasma anti-heparin activity and platelet survival time in coronary disease. Am Heart J 99, 438-442, 1980.

449. Stein L, Beraud JJ, Morisette M, DaLuz P, Weil MH: Pulmonary edema during volume infusion. Circulation 52, 483-489, 1975.
450. Stein TP, Leskiw MJ, Wallace HW: Measurement of half-life of human plasma fibrinogen. Am J Physiol 234, E504-E510, 1978.
451. Sterling K: The turnover rate of serum albumin in man as measured by I-131-tagged albumin. J Clin Invest 30, 1228-1237, 1951.
452. Sternlieb J, Morell AG, Tucker WD, Greene MW, Scheinberg JH: The incorporation of copper into ceruloplasmin in vivo: studies with copper 64 and copper 67. J Clin Invest 40, 1834-1840, 1961.
453. Stevenson GT: Immunoglobulins. In: Structure and function of plasma proteins. AC Allison (Ed), Plenum Press, London, 1974, 223-264.
454. Stone MJ, Willerson JT, Gomez-Sanchez CE, Waterman MR: Radio-immunoassay of myoglobin in human serum. Results in patients with acute myocardial infarction. J Clin Invest 56, 1334-1339, 1975.
455. Strandjord PE, Thomas KE, White LP: Studies on isocitric and lactic dehydrogenases in experimental myocardial infarction. J Clin Invest 38, 2111-2118, 1959.
456. Strober W, Wochner RD, Barlow MH, McFarlin DE, Waldmann TA: Immunoglobulin metabolism in Ataxia Telangiectasia. J Clin Invest 47, 1905-1915, 1968.
457. Suttie JW, McTigue J, Larson AE, Wallin R: Biosynthesis of prothrombin complex proteins. Ann NY Acad Sci 370, 271-280, 1981.
458. Sylvén C: The kinetics of myoglobin in old volunteers and in patients with acute myocardial infarction. Scand J Clin Lab Invest 38, 561-565, 1978.
459. Szabó G, Magyar Z: Intracellular enzymes in serum, lymph and urine after renal ischemia: Lymphology 7, 13-22, 1974.
460. Szabó G: Movement of proteins into blood capillaries. In: Ergebnisse der Angiologie. Basic Lymphology, Földi M (Ed). Stuttgart, FK Schattauer Verlag, 1976, 31-50.
461. Szabó G, Magyar Z: The relationship between tissue fluid and lymph II. Enzymes in tissue fluid and lymph. Lymphology 11, 101-105, 1978.
462. Szabó G: Enzymes in tissue fluid and peripheral lymph. Lymphology 11, 147-155, 1978.
463. Szabó G, Magyar Z: Biochemical changes in the body fluids after ischemic tissue injury. Lymphology 13, 74-77, 1980.
464. Takeda Y, Reeve EB: Studies of the metabolism and distribution of albumin with autologous I-131-albumin in healthy men. J Lab Clin Med 61, 183-202, 1963.
465. Takeda Y: Studies on the metabolism and distribution of fibrinogen in healthy men with autologous 125-I-labelled fibrinogen. J Clin Invest 45, 103-111, 1966.
466. Takeda Y: Studies on the metabolism and distribution of fibrinogen in patients with rheumatoid arthritis. J Lab Clin Med 69, 624-633, 1967.
467. Takeda Y, Chen AY: Fibrinogen metabolism and distribution in patients with the nephrotic syndrome. J Lab Clin Med 70, 678-685, 1967.
468. Takeda Y, Chen AY: Studies of the metabolism and distribution of fibrinogen in patients with hemophilia A. J Clin Invest 46, 1979-1985, 1967.
469. Takeda Y: Studies of the metabolism and distribution of prothrombin in healthy men with homologous 125-I-prothrombin. Thromb Diath Haemorrh 27, 472-489, 1972.
470. Takeda Y, Takeuchi T: Studies of fibrinogen metabolism in healthy and hypertensive female subjects wwith the use of autologous I-125-fibrinogen. Thromb Haemostas (Stuttg) 39, 39-45, 1978.
472. Tavill AS, Hoffenberg R: Turnover of plasma proteins. In: Structure and function of plasma proteins, vol 2. AC Allison (ed), Plenum Press, New

York, 1976, 107-188.

473. Taylor AE, Granger DN, Brace RA: Analysis of lymphatic flux data I. Estimation of the reflection coefficient and permeability-surface area product for total protein. Microvasc Res 13, 297-313, 1977.

474. Teorell T: Kinetics of distribution of substances administered to the body. I The extravascular modes of administration. Arch Int Pharmacodyn Ther 57, 205-240, 1937.

475. Theiss W, Wirtzfeld W: Coagulation studies and rheological considerations in a subsample of patients pertaining to the European trial of streptokinase in acute myocardial infarction. Acta Med Scand, Suppl 648, 97-104, 1981.

476. Thompson PL, Fletcher EE, Katavatis V: Enzymatic indices of myocardial necrosis; influence on short- and long-term prognosis after myocardial infarction. Circulation 59, 113-119, 1979.

477. Thornburg RW, Day JF, Baynes JW, Thorpe SR: Carbohydrate-mediated clearance of immune complexes from the circulation - a role for galactose residues in the hepatic uptake of IgG-antigen complexes. J Biol Chem 255, 6820-6825, 1980.

478. Thorstensson A, Sjödin B, Tesch P, Karlsson J: Actomyosin ATPase, Myokinase, CPK, and LDH in human fast and slow twitch muscle fibres. Acta Physiol Scand 99, 225-229, 1977.

479. Tommasini G, Presta M: Prediction of infarct size by enzymatic techniques; modification of a method and clinical application. Br heart J 42, 326-332, 1979.

480. Tota B: On the regional metabolism of beef heart ventricles. Acta Physiol Scand 87, 289-295, 1973.

481. Trahern CA, Brewster GJ, Krauth GH, Bigham DA: Clinical assessment of serum myosin light chains in the diagnosis of acute myocardial infarction. Am J Cardiol 41, 641-645, 1978.

482. Tytgat GN, Collen D, Verstraete M: Metabolism of fibrinogen in cirrhosis of the liver. J Clin Invest 50, 1690-1701, 1971.

483. Ussing HH: The interpretation of tracer fluxes in terms of membrane structure. Quart Rev Biophys 1, 365-376, 1969.

484. Vahlquist A, Peterson PA, Wibell L: Metabolism of the vitamin A transporting protein complex I. Turnover studies in normal persons and in patients with chronic renal failure. Eur J Clin Invest 3, 352-362, 1973.

485. Van Beaumont W, Greenleaf JE, Juhos L: Disproportional changes in hematocrit, plasma volume and proteins during exercise and bed rest. J Appl Physiol 33, 55-61, 1972.

486. Van Beaumont W, Rochelle RH: Erythrocyte volume stability with plasma osmolarity changes in excercising man. Proc Soc Exp Biol Med 145, 240-243, 1974.

487. Van der Laarse A: On the multiple polarographic measurement of myocardial oxygen tension. Thesis, Amsterdam, 1978.

488. Van der Laarse A, Hollaar L, van der Valk LJM, Witteveen SAGJ: Enzyme release from and enzyme depletion in rat heart cell cultures during anoxia. J Mol Med 3, 123-131, 1978.

489. Van der Laarse A, Hollaar L, Kokshoorn LJM, Witteveen SAGJ: The activity of cardio-specific isoenzymes of creatine phosphokinase and lactate dehydrogenase in monolayer cultures of neonatal rat heart cells. J Mol Cell Cardiol 11, 501-510, 1979.

490. Van der Laarse A, Hollaar L, Van der Valk JM: Release of alpha-hydroxybutyrate dehydrogenase from neonatal rat heart cell cultures exposed to anoxia and reoxygenation. Comparison with impairment of structure and function of damaged cardiac cells. Cardiovasc Res 13, 345-353, 1979.

491. Van der Laarse A: Quantification of anoxia-induced cell damage in rat

heart cell cultures using enzymatic, histologic and contractile perform-ance techniques. In: Quantification of myocardial ischemia. H Kreuzer, WW Parmley, P Rentrop, HW Heiss (Eds). New York, Gerhard Witzstrock Publ House, 1980, 461-471.

492. Van der Laarse A, Dijkshoorn NJ, Hollaar L, Caspers T: The (iso)-enzyme activities of lactate dehydrogenase, alpha-hydroxybutyrate dehydrogenase, creatine kinase and aspartate aminotransferase in human myocardial biop-sies and autopsies. Clin Chim Acta, 104, 381-391, 1980.

493. Van der Laarse A, Davids HA, Hollaar L, Hermens WT: Enhanced release of mitochondrial aspartate aminotransferase (mAST) from anoxic heart cell cultures during reoxygenation. Comparison to plasma mAST levels in pa-tients after acute myocardial infarction and after cardiac surgery. Car-diovasc Res 15, 11-20, 1981.

495. Van der Meer J, Hemker HC, Loeliger EA: Pharmacological aspects of vi-tamin K1. A clinical and experimental study in man. Thrombos Diathes Haemorrh Suppl 29, 1968.

496. Van Dieijen-Visser MP: Behaviour of tissue enzymes in the circulation. Thesis, Meppel, 1981.

497. Van Furth R, Cohn ZA, Hirsch JG, Humphrey JH, Spector WG, Langevoort HL: The mononuclear phagocyte system; a new classification of macrophages, monocytes and their precursor cells. Bull Wld Hlth Org 46, 845-852, 1972.

498. Van Oosterom AT, Mattie H, Hermens WT, Veltkamp JJ: The influence of the thyroid function on the metabolic rate of prothrombin, factor VII, and factor X in the rat. Thromb Haemostas (Stuttg) 35, 607-619, 1976.

499. Van Zile J, Henderson LA, Baynes JW, Thorpe SR: 3H-Raffinose, a novel radioactive label for determining organ sites of catabolism of proteins in the circulation. J Biol Chem 254, 3547-3553, 1979.

500. Veltkamp JJ, Loeliger EA, Hemker HC: The biological half-time of Hageman factor. Thromb Diath Haemorrh 13, 1-7, 1965.

501. Veress B, Kerenyi T, Hüttner J, Jellinek H: The phases of muscle necro-sis. J Path Bact 92, 511-517, 1966.

502. Versavel C, Jousset-Stevenat B, Lebreton de Vonne T, Besnard J-C, Mouray H: Le métabolisme des alpha macroglobulines du lapin: étude de la demi-vie. CRBiol (Paris) 30 septembre, 245-247, 1976.

503. Visser MP: The two-compartment circulatory model used for enzymatic in-farct quantitation. Circ Res 42, 877-879, 1978.

504. Visser MP, Krill MTA, Boumans ML, Willems GM, Hermens WT: Selection of marker enzymes for the quantitation of tissue damage. Eur Heart J 2, Suppl A, 22, 1981.

505. Visser MP, Krill MTA, Muijtjens AMM, Willems GM, Hermens WT: Distribution of enzymes in dog heart and liver. Significance for assessment of tissue damage from data on plasma enzyme activities. Clin Chem 27, 1845-1850, 1981.

506. Visser MP, Krill MTA, Willems GM, Hermens WT: Selection of a suitable circulatory model for the plasma clearance and distribution of cardiac enzymes in the dog. Cardiovasc Res 15, 35-42, 1981.

507. Visser MP, Krill MTA, Willems GM, Hermens WT: Plasma volume determination by use of enzyme dilution in the dog. Lab Animals 16, 248-255, 1982.

508. Vitek F, Bianchi R, Donato L: The study of distribution and catabolism of labeled serum albumin by means of analog computer technique. J Nucl Biol Med 10, 121-130, 1966.

509. Volk P: Myoglobin in the serum after myocardial infarction. München Med Wschr 115, 2122-2128, 1973.

510. Volwiler W, Goldsworthy PD, McMartin MP, Wood PA, Mackay JR, Fremont-Smith K: Biosynthetic determination with radioactive sulfur of turnover rates of various plasma proteins in normal and cirrhotic man. J Clin

Invest 34, 1126-1146, 1955.
511. Wakim KG, Fleisher GA: The fate of enzymes in body fluids - an experimental study II. Disappearance rates of glutamic - oxalacetic transaminase I under various conditions. J Lab Clin Med 61, 86-97, 1963.
512. Wakim KG, Fleisher GA: The fate of enzymes in body fluids - an experimental study IV. Relationship of the reticulo-endothelial system to activities and disappearance rates of various enzymes. J Lab Clin Med 61, 107-119, 1963.
513. Waldmann TA, Strober W: Metabolism of immunoglobulins. Progr Allergy 13, 1-110, 1969.
514. Waldmann TA, Iio A, Ogawa M, McIntyre OR, Strober W: The metabolism of IgE. Studies in normal individuals and in a patient with IgE myeoloma. J Immunol 117, 1139-1144, 1976.
515. Wallevik K: In vivo structure and stability of serum albumin in relation to its normal catabolism. Acta Physiol Scand, suppl 471, 1-56, 1979.
516. Walls WD, Losowsky MS: Plasma fibrin stabilising factor (FSF) activity in normal subjects and patients with chronic lever disease. Thromb Diathes Haemorrh 21, 21-27, 1969.
517. Wasserman K, Mayerson HS: Exchange of albumin between plasma and lymph. Am J Physiol 165, 15-26, 1951.
518. Weiser PC, Grande F: Estimation of fluid shifts and protein permeability during pulmonary edemagenesis. Am J Physiol 226, 1028-1034, 1974.
519. Weisman S, Goldsmith B, Winzler R, Lepper MH: Turnover of plasma orosomucoid in man. J Lab Clin Med 57, 7-15, 1961.
520. Wells JV: Immunoglobulins: biosynthesis and metabolism. In: Basic and clinical immunology. HH Fudenberg (Ed), Los Altos (Calif.), Lange, 1980, third ed, 64-78.
521. Welman E, Selwyn AP, Peters TJ, Colbeck JF, Fox KM: Plasma lysosomal enzyme activity in acute myocardial infarction. Cardiovasc Res 12, 99-105, 1978.
522. Werner M: Serum protein changes during the acute phase reaction. Clin Chim Acta 25, 299-305, 1969.
523. Wetterfors J: Catabolism and distribution of serum-ablumin in the dog. An experimental study with homologous 131-I-albumin. Acta Med Scand 177, 243-256, 1965.
524. Wevers RA, Desling M, Klein Gebbink JAG, Soons JBJ: Post-synthetic changes in creatine kinase isoenzymes (EC 2.7.3.2). Clin Chim Acta 86, 323-327, 1978.
525. Wevers RA, Mul-Steinbusch MWFJ, Soons JBJ: Mitochondrial CK (EC 2.7.3.2) in the human heart. Clin Chim Acta 101, 103-111, 1980.
526. Wiederhielm CA: Dynamics of capillary fluid exchange. A nonlinear computer simulation. Microvasc Res 18, 48-82, 1979.
527. Willems GM, Muijtjens AMM, Lambi FHH, Hermens WT: Estimation of circulatory parameters in patients with acute myocardial infarction. Significance for calculation of enzymatic infarct size. Cardiovasc Res 13, 578-587, 1979.
528. Willems GM, Visser MP, Krill MTA, Hermens WT: Quantitative analysis of plasma enzyme levels based upon simultaneous determination of different enzymes. Cardiovasc Res 16, 120-131, 1982.
529. Wissenschaftlichte Tabellen Geigy: Hämatologie und Humangenetik, (Ciba-Geigy) 8. Auflage, Basel, 1979.
530. Witteveen SAGJ, Hermens WT, Hemker HC, Hollaar L: Quantitation of enzyme release from infarcted heart muscle. In: Ischemic heart disease. JH de Haas, HC Hemker, HA Snellen (Eds). Leiden, Univ Press, 1970, 36-42.
531. Witteveen SAGJ: Assessment of the extent of a myocardial infarction on the basis of plasma enzyme levels. Thesis, Leiden, 1972.

532. Witteveen SAGJ, Hemker HC, Hollaar L, Hermens WT: Quantitation of infarct size in man by means of plasma enzyme levels. Br Heart J $\underline{37}$, 795-803, 1975.

533. Wochner RD: Hypercatabolism of normal IgG; an unexplained immunoglobulin abnormality in the connective tissue diseases. J Clin Invest $\underline{49}$, 454-464, 1970.

534. Wochner RD, Spilberg J, Iio A, Liem HH, Muller-Eberhard U: Hemopexin metabolism in sickle-cell disease, porphyrias and control subjects - effects of heme injection. New Eng J Med $\underline{290}$, 822-826, 1974.

535. Wohlgemuth J: Über eine neue Methode zur quantitativen Bestimmung des diastatischen Ferments. Biochem Z $\underline{9}$, 1-9, 1908.

536. Wróblewski F, LaDue JS: Serum glutamic oxaloacetic transaminase activity as an index of liver cell injury; a preliminary report. Ann Intern Med $\underline{43}$, 345-360, 1955.

537. Yasmineh WG, Pyle RB, Hanson NQ, Hultman BK: Creatine kinase isoenzymes in baboon tissues and organs. Clin Chem $\underline{22}$, 63-66, 1976.

538. Yasmineh WG, Ibrahim GA, Abbasnezhad M, Awad EA: Isoenzyme distribution of creatine kinase and lactate dehydrogenase in serum and skeletal muscle in Duchenne muscular dystrophy, collagen disease and other muscular disorders. Clin Chem $\underline{24}$, 1985-1989, 1978.

539. Zak R, Martin AF, Blough R: Assessment of protein turnover by use of radioisotopic tracers. Physiol Rev $\underline{59}$, 407-447, 1979.

540. Zeineh RA, Kukral JC: The turnover rate of orosomucoid in burned patients. J Trauma $\underline{10}$, 493-498, 1970.

541. Zierler KL: Muscle membrane as a dynamic structure and its permeability to aldolase. Ann NY Acad Sci $\underline{75}$, 227-234, 1958.